Manual of
Oxygen Therapy

Manual of Oxygen Therapy

Editors

Kapil Zirpe
MD (Chest) FCCM FICCM
Head
Department of Neuro Critical Care
Ruby Hall Clinic, Grant Medical Foundation
Pune, Maharashtra, India

Subhal B Dixit
MD (Med) IDCCM FCCM FICCM FICP
Director
Department of Critical Care
Sanjeevan Hospital
Pune, Maharashtra, India

Atul P Kulkarni
MD (Anesthesiology) FISCCM PGDHHM FICCM
Professor and Head
Division of Critical Care Medicine
Department of Anesthesiology, Critical Care and Pain
Tata Memorial Hospital
Homi Bhabha National Institute
Mumbai, Maharashtra, India

Associate Editors

Shilpushp Bhosale
DM (Critical Care Medicine) Fellowship Pediatric
Critical Care (Canada)
Professor
Division of Critical Care Medicine
Department of Anesthesiology
Critical Care and Pain Tata Memorial Centre
Homi Bhabha National Institute
Mumbai, Maharashtra, India

Khalid Ismail Khatib
MD (Medicine) FICCM FICP
Professor
Department of Medicine
SKN Medical College
Pune, Maharashtra, India

Forewords

Ashish K Khanna, BD Kadam

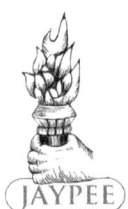

JAYPEE BROTHERS MEDICAL PUBLISHERS
The Health Sciences Publisher
New Delhi | London

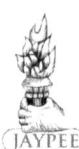

Jaypee Brothers Medical Publishers (P) Ltd

Headquarters

Jaypee Brothers Medical Publishers (P) Ltd
EMCA House, 23/23-B
Ansari Road, Daryaganj
New Delhi 110 002, India
Landline: +91-11-23272143, +91-11-23272703
+91-11-23282021, +91-11-23245672
Email: jaypee@jaypeebrothers.com

Corporate Office

Jaypee Brothers Medical Publishers (P) Ltd
4838/24, Ansari Road, Daryaganj
New Delhi 110 002, India
Phone: +91-11-43574357
Fax: +91-11-43574314
Email: jaypee@jaypeebrothers.com

Overseas Office

JP Medical Ltd
83 Victoria Street, London
SW1H 0HW (UK)
Phone: +44 20 3170 8910
Fax: +44 (0)20 3008 6180
Email: info@jpmedpub.com

Website: www.jaypeebrothers.com
Website: www.jaypeedigital.com

© 2022, Jaypee Brothers Medical Publishers

The views and opinions expressed in this book are solely those of the original contributor(s)/author(s) and do not necessarily represent those of editor(s) or publisher of the book.

All rights reserved. No part of this publication may be reproduced, stored or transmitted in any form or by any means, electronic, mechanical, photocopying, recording or otherwise, without the prior permission in writing of the publishers.

All brand names and product names used in this book are trade names, service marks, trademarks or registered trademarks of their respective owners. The publisher is not associated with any product or vendor mentioned in this book.

Medical knowledge and practice change constantly. This book is designed to provide accurate, authoritative information about the subject matter in question. However, readers are advised to check the most current information available on procedures included and check information from the manufacturer of each product to be administered, to verify the recommended dose, formula, method and duration of administration, adverse effects and contraindications. It is the responsibility of the practitioner to take all appropriate safety precautions. Neither the publisher nor the author(s)/editor(s) assume any liability for any injury and/or damage to persons or property arising from or related to use of material in this book.

This book is sold on the understanding that the publisher is not engaged in providing professional medical services. If such advice or services are required, the services of a competent medical professional should be sought.

Every effort has been made where necessary to contact holders of copyright to obtain permission to reproduce copyright material. If any have been inadvertently overlooked, the publisher will be pleased to make the necessary arrangements at the first opportunity. The **CD/DVD-ROM** (if any) provided in the sealed envelope with this book is complimentary and free of cost. **Not meant for sale.**

Inquiries for bulk sales may be solicited at: jaypee@jaypeebrothers.com

Manual of Oxygen Therapy

First Edition: **2022**

ISBN: 978-93-5465-655-2

Contributors

Abhijit Deshmukh
MBBS TDD IDCCM
Consultant In-Charge
Neuro Trauma Unit
Ruby Hall Clinic
Pune, Maharashtra, India

Apoorva Tiwari MBBS
Attending Consultant
Department of Critical Care
Artemis Hospital
Gurugram, Haryana, India

Atul P Kulkarni
MD (Anesthesiology) FISCCM
PGDHHM FICCM
Professor and Head
Division of Critical Care
Medicine
Department of Anesthesiology,
Critical Care and Pain
Tata Memorial Hospital
Homi Bhabha National Institute
Mumbai, Maharashtra, India

Balkrishan Nimavat
MD DNB FNB IDCCM EDIC EDAIC
Consultant
Department of Critical Care
Sir HN Reliance Hospital
Mumbai, Maharashtra, India

Beena Daniel MBBS DA
Consultant Intensivist
Department of
Critical Care Medicine
Medicover Hospitals
Aurangabad, Maharashtra,
India

Deeksha Singh Tomar
DA IDCCM IFCCM EDIC
Consultant
Department of Critical Care
Narayana Superspecialty
Hospital
Gurugram, Haryana, India

Deepak Govil
MD EDIC FICCM FCCM
Director, Critical Care
Institute of Critical Care and
Anesthesia
Medanta—the Medicity
Gurugram, Haryana, India

Deepu K Peter
MD DNB (Resp Med)
Assistant Professor
Department of Pulmonary
Medicine
Command Hospital (NC)
Udhampur, Jammu and
Kashmir, India

Deven Juneja
DNB FNB EDIC FCCP IFCCM FCCM
Director
Department of Institute of
Critical Care Medicine
Max Super Specialty Hospital
New Delhi, India

Divya Pal MD FNB
Consultant
Department of Critical Care
Medicine
Medanta—the Medicity
Gurugram, Haryana, India

Gunjan Chanchalani
MD IFCCM FNB FICCM EDICM
Chief Intensivist
Department of Critical Care
KJ Somaiya Hospital and
Research Centre
Mumbai, Maharashtra, India

Harjit Dumra MD (Medicine)
Head
Department of Critical Care
Medicine
Sterling Hospital
Ahmedabad, Gujarat, India

Inderpaul Singh Sehgal
Assistant Professor
Department of Pulmonary
Medicine
Postgraduate Institute of
Medical Education and
Research
Chandigarh, India

Jeetendra Sharma
MD IDCCM IFCCM FICCM
Chief (Critical Care Medicine)
and Chief (Medical Quality)
Artemis Hospital
Gurugram, Haryana, India

Jitin Sharma
MD (Anesthesiology)
Senior Consultant
Department of Critical Care
Medicine
BLK MAX Superspeciality
Hospital
New Delhi, India

Contributors

Kanwalpreet Sodhi
DA DNB IDCCM EDIC
Director and Head
Department of Critical Care
Deep Hospital
Ludhiana, Punjab, India

Kapil Borawake
DNB IDCCM FICCM
Director
Department of Intensive Care
and General Medicine
Vishwaraj Hospital and
Research Centre
Pune, Maharashtra, India

Kapil Zirpe
MD (Chest) FCCM FICCM
Head
Department of Neuro Critical
Care
Ruby Hall Clinic, Grant Medical
Foundation
Pune, Maharashtra, India

Khalid Ismail Khatib
MD (Medicine) FICCM FICP
Professor
Department of Medicine
SKN Medical College
Pune, Maharashtra, India

**Kiran Raghavendra
Asrnanna** MD (DrNB)
Senior Trainee
Department of Critical Care
Virinchi Hospitals
Hyderabad, Telangana, India

Maitree Pandey
MD (Anesthesiology)
Director Professor and Head
Department of Anesthesiology
and Critical Care
Lady Hardinge Medical College
New Delhi, India

Malini Joshi
MD (Anesthesiology)
Professor
Department of Anesthesiology,
Critical Care and Pain
Tata Memorial Centre
Homi Bhabha National Institute
Mumbai, Maharashtra, India

Manender Kumar
MD (Anesthesia) PDCC (Cardiac
Anesthesia & Critical Care)
Additional Director
Department of Cardiac
Anesthesia
Fortis Hospital
Ludhiana, Punjab, India

Mansi Dandnaik
MD IDCCM EDICM
Consultant
Department of Critical Care
Medicine
Sterling Hospital
Ahmedabad, Gujarat, India

Prajakta Pote MBBS DNB
(Anesthesia) IDCCM IFCCM
Fellowship in Neurocritical Care
Fellowship in Critical
Care Ultrasound
Senior Consultant
Department of
Neurotrauma Unit
Ruby Hall Clinic
Pune, Maharashtra, India

Prashant Nasa MD FNB
(Critical Care Medicine) EDICM
SCE-Acute Medicine
Head
Department of Critical Care
Medicine
NMC Specialty Hospital
Dubai, UAE

Rahul Pandit MD FCICM FJFICM
FCCP EDIC IFCCM DA
Director (Critical Care)
Fortis Hospital
Mumbai, Maharashtra, India

Rajesh Chandra MD IDCCM
DNB SS Trainee
Department of Critical Care
Medicine
Medanta Hospital
Ranchi, Jharkhand, India

Rajesh Pande
MD PDCC FICCM FCCM
Senior Director and Head
Department of Critical Care
Medicine
BLK-Max Super Specialty
Hospital
New Delhi, India

Robin Choudhary
MD (Resp Med)
Senior Resident
Department of Pulmonary
Medicine
Army Institute of Cardio-
Thoracic Sciences (AICTS)
Pune, Maharashtra, India

Sachin Gupta MD IDCCM
IFCCM EDIC FCCM FICCM
Director
Department of Critical Care
Narayana Superspecialty
Hospital
Gurugram, Haryana, India

Sahil Kataria DNB
Fellow
Institute of Critical Care
Medicine
Max Super Specialty Hospital
New Delhi, India

Contributors

Sameer V Kulkarni
MD (Anes) IDCCM
Professor
Department of Anesthesia
Smt Kashibai Navale Medical College
Pune, Maharashtra, India

Santanu Bagchi
MD FNB
Consultant
Critical Care Medicine
Tata Medical Center
Kolkata, West Bengal, India

Shabeer Ahmed Khan
MD (DrNB)
Senior Trainee
Department of Critical Care
Virinchi Hospitals
Hyderabad, Telangana, India

Shikha Sahi
MBBS MD IFCCM
Consultant (Critical Care)
Artemis Hospital
Gurugram, Haryana, India

Shilpushp Bhosale DM
(Critical Care Medicine) Fellowship
Pediatric Critical Care (Canada)
Professor
Division of Critical Care Medicine
Department of Anesthesiology,
Critical Care and Pain
Tata Memorial Centre
Homi Bhabha National Institute
Mumbai, Maharashtra, India

Shrikant Sahasrabudhe
MD (Chest) IDCCM TDD
Director and Head
Senior Consultant
Pulmonologist and
Critical Care Specialist
Department of Pulmonology
and Critical Care Medicine
Medicover Hospitals
Aurangabad, Maharashtra, India
Examiner and Teacher for
IDCCM/CTCCM

Sonali Ghosh MBBS DCH
MRCPCH (UK) IDPCCM
Senior Consultant
Pediatrics and In-charge
PICU, QRG Superspecialty Hospital
Faridabad, Haryana, India

Srinivas Samavedam MD
DNB FRCP FNB EDIC DMLE FICCM MBA
Head and Medical Director
Department of Critical Care
Virinchi Hospitals
Hyderabad, Telangana, India

Subhal B Dixit MD (Med)
IDCCM FCCM FICCM FICP
Director
Department of Critical Care
Sanjeevan Hospital
Pune, Maharashtra, India

Sunil Amin MBBS MD IDCCM
Consultant Chest Physician and Intensivist
Department of Critical Care
Param Multispecialty and ICU
Surat, Gujarat, India

Supradip Ghosh MBBS DNB
(Internal Medicine) MRCP (UK) EDIC FICCM
Director and Head
Critical Care Medicine
Fortis Escorts Hospital
Faridabad, Haryana, India

Tapas Kumar Sahoo
MD FNB FICCM FCCP EDIC MBA
Senior Consultant and Head
Department of Critical
Care Medicine
Medanta Hospital
Ranchi, Jharkhand, India

Ujwala Mhatre Ahluwalia
MBBS DA DNB IFCCM IDCCM
Senior Consultant (Critical Care)
Ramkrishna Care Hospital
Raipur, Chhattisgarh, India

Vikas Marwah
MD (Resp Med) SCE (RCP) UK
Professor and Head
Department of Pulmonary Medicine
Army Institute of Cardio-Thoracic Sciences (AICTS)
Pune, Maharashtra, India

Vikram Damaraju MD DM
Senior Resident
Department of Pulmonary Medicine
Postgraduate Institute
of Medical Education
and Research
Chandigarh, India

Foreword

Oxygen is a much-utilized 'medication' in the inpatient environment. Whether the operating room, the intensive care unit or other acute care areas, most have access to this easily available agent. In fact, oxygen is the one thing that we turn to as a reflex action, whenever our patients are in a crisis. However, oxygen is also a drug, and like all other pharmacological interventions has a therapeutic window and potential adverse effects. Most commonly, we end up placing patients who leave the post-anesthesia care unit (PACU) or the emergency room or ICU on a few liters of oxygen for comfort or to keep their oxygen saturation numbers looking satisfactory. This practice is rather dangerous and may mask respiratory distress, specifically hypoventilation in situations where spontaneously breathing patients have an inadequate respiratory drive and with no measures of ventilation to guide therapy. Similarly, the use of high-inspired oxygen in ventilated ICU patients has the potential for free radical damage and absorption atelectasis, both often missed because of subtle early presentation. The need to understand, physiology, pharmacology, physics, and delivery of oxygen in a precise manner is paramount for improving patient outcomes. Unfortunately, there is a paucity of education around the use of this life-saving agent, even though all of us use it nearly every single day, we work in the hospital.

It is a pleasure to see this the first edition of the *Manual of Oxygen Therapy*, edited by three stalwarts in critical care and acute care medicine. I have known the editors, Dr(s) Kapil Zirpe, Subhal Dixit, and Atul P Kulkarni through their work in the field, and tremendous contributions to the Indian Society of Critical Care Medicine (ISCCM). It is not a surprise to me that they have put together an excellent compilation of authors and knowledge areas in this manual. The text itself is nicely divided into four sections that range from handling medical oxygen as a gas, monitoring the use of oxygen in the context of the physiology of gas exchange, delivery devices, toxicity, and therapy for individualized disease states. This will serve as a source of ready reference for the experienced clinicians, and a rich textbook for the medical students and trainees in medicine or paramedical fields. My very best wishes to this team, and congratulations on publishing this much-needed work that will benefit all of us.

Ashish K Khanna
MD FCCP FCCM FASA
Associate Professor, Vice-Chair for Research
Director, Perioperative Outcomes and Informatics Collaborative (POIC)
Department of Anesthesiology, Section on Critical Care Medicine
Wake Forest University School of Medicine
Atrium Health Wake Forest Baptist Medical Center
Winston-Salem, NC, USA 27106

Foreword

It gives me great pleasure to write foreword for *Manual of Oxygen Therapy*. All the contributors to this book are critical care specialists, who deal with oxygen day-in and day-out.

They have put all their experience in this book and made it of practical utility than theoretical knowledge.

Oxygen is abundant in the atmosphere. We realize its importance only when it is most necessary for our survival. In my experience, I realized why oxygen is called *Pranavayu* in most of the vernacular languages, you remember it when you need it in your life.

After visiting Leh, I realized that even when walking for 10 steps, my colleagues and I cannot breathe easily. This was my first experience of hypoxia. It feels as though someone is trying to stop your breathing. It can be treated with oxygen inhalation and adequate bed rest. This is when you realize the importance of oxygen.

A second experience, I had was with Corona epidemic. The press reported that elderly people were giving up their oxygen beds for the sake of a young person. This was because oxygen was in short supply and patients were running from pillar to post of every hospital to get oxygen beds to save themselves or their relatives. Oxygen audit came into existence after this episode. Everyone realized oxygen was the most important resource in dealing with Corona epidemic.

If we look at the history of oxygen, we realize that oxygen was discovered by Carl Wilhelm Scheele in 1771 and named by Antoine Lavoisier as oxygen. Oxygen is atomic number 8. It is a highly reactive nonmetal oxidizing agent. It is present in the earth's atmosphere to the tune of 20.95%. Its stable compound is a di-oxygen molecule. Oxygen is used as therapy when it is supplied as a supplement to breathe in addition to air for hypoxemia. It can be utilized in various formats such as home oxygen therapy, hyperbaric oxygen therapy, hospital-based oxygen therapy, and extracorporeal membrane oxygenation (ECMO). It is an essential medicine classified by WHO. Normally, saturation of oxygen in the body is to the tune of 94–96%, however in COPD patients, it can be 88–92%. One can start oxygen at saturation of less than 90% and stop the same above 96%. Yes, there are contraindications to oxygen therapy such as paraquat poisoning, bleomycin, aspiration, and sepsis to avoid hyperoxia. Its pathophysiological effects include absorption atelectasis, airway inflammation, CNS effects, CO_2 retention, pulmonary vascular and systematic vasoconstriction when given more than demand. Hence oxygen therapy is to be used judiciously for saving a patient's life.

The present manual on oxygen therapy is a comprehensive effort to delineate various aspects of oxygen therapy. Dr Kapil Zirpe, Dr Subhal B Dixit, Dr Atul P Kulkarni, and their colleagues have certainly made a valuable contribution to society with this effort.

Section 1 of this book deals with the basics of oxygen purity, storage distribution, and safety of oxygen. With multiple incidents of fires in hospitals claiming lives, safety becomes the most critical aspect. It is equally important to distribute oxygen to multiple wards and the ICU to justify oxygen usage.

Section 2 of the book talks about the physiological effects of oxygen therapy and the basics of gas exchange. This gives us insights into oxygen therapy. It also speaks about targets in oxygen therapy and preventing oxygen toxicity. This section will enable physicians to use oxygen as a pharmaceutical agent with the appropriate understanding of its limitations and implications, including interpretation of blood gas analysis, oxygen dissociation curves, and monitoring by pulseoxymetry and its limitations.

Section 3 describes various oxygen delivery systems. During COVID epidemic, role of high flow oxygen therapy became the therapy of choice. Before this mode was underutilized. It is explained in this chapter how to use various delivery systems, ranging from a nasal catheter to intubation and ventilator in a graduated manner, without creating unnecessary and unsupervised oxygen toxicity.

Final section 4 describes the effect of hypoxia on various organ systems and how to revert it by using oxygen therapy. The mechanism of this therapy is described in detail. Oxygen therapy has to be utilized in light of underlying comorbidity and underlying lung or any other systematic disorder. Normal versus diseased lung ventilation for hypoxemia is different. Furthermore diseases such as ARDS, COPD, myocardial infarction, and stroke will change various aspects of oxygen therapy.

Thus this book will be a one-stop guide for oxygen therapy in a variety of disorders for physicians. This book should be a reference book in every place where oxygen therapy is being delivered as it will guide physicians to get optimal results from oxygen therapy. I congratulate editors and team for this wonderful venture.

BD Kadam
Professor Medicine Emeritus
BJ Government Medical College
Pune, Maharashtra, India
Chairman, COVID-19 Task Force, Pune Division
Master Teacher Awardee By Association of Physicians of India (API)

Preface

Dear Friends, it gives us great pleasure in presenting to you this *Manual of Oxygen Therapy*. Ongoing COVID-19 pandemic has brought up number of respiratory issues. Many of us are unaware of administrative hard-work that is required, the detailed planning this entails in getting a small innocuous looking cylinder at the patient's bedside. Many doctors who are normally not called upon to provide oxygen therapy to patients in their routine clinical activities were forced to look after patients who were not only sick, but were requiring high fraction of inspired oxygen, during this unusual situation. Although oxygen therapy may be common in the various settings in hospital, it is used quite rarely at home under normal circumstances. The pandemic-forced patients to use oxygen at home, when clinicians were forced to discharge patients on oxygen therapy.

We felt that there is a lack of a source which will provide detailed information about how oxygen is stored, how it piped to the bedside of the intended recipient and how it should be administered. This manual of oxygen therapy is our attempt to provide this, and other information regarding its appropriate use, devices which are used deliver oxygen to the patient and complications associated with oxygen therapy. Thus, our main purpose in writing this manual was to spread knowledge among non-acute care practicing clinicians, critical care trainee and paramedics. This book will be a good source of ready reference.

While preparing the table of contents, we have tried to cover topics ranging from differences between industrial and medical gas, medical gas pipeline designs physiology gas exchange, to oxygen therapy targeted towards specific diseases. The contributions have come from experts in the subject and from all corners of India.

This book is user-friendly and provides information in structured manner. We hope the readers will enjoy reading this book as much as loved planning, designing and writing it. It is also our fervent hope that it proves handy in day-to-day practice of the busy clinicians, juniors and seniors alike.

Best wishes!

Kapil Zirpe
Subhal B Dixit
Atul P Kulkarni

Contents

SECTION 1: Basic Facts of Oxygen

1. **Industrial and Medical Oxygen Production and Differences** 3
   Balkrishna Nimavat, Abhijit Deshmukh, Kapil Zirpe

2. **Medical Piped Gas Structure, Design, and Safety Systems** 8
   Prajakta Pote, Kapil Zirpe

3. **Medical Compressed Gas Cylinder: Handling and Use** 16
   Vikas Marwah, Deepu K Peter, Robin Choudhary

4. **Cryogenic Liquid Medical Oxygen** 22
   Shikha Sahi, Apoorva Tiwari, Jeetendra Sharma

5. **Oxygen Concentrators** 32
   Khalid Ismail Khatib, Sameer V Kulkarni, Subhal B Dixit

6. **Oxygen Hazards and Safety** 35
   Deven Juneja, Prashant Nasa, Sahil Kataria

7. **Oxygen Audit** 40
   Rahul Pandit

SECTION 2: Physiology and Monitoring of Oxygen Therapy

8. **Physiology of Gas Exchange** 47
   Shilpushp Bhosale, Malini Joshi, Atul P Kulkarni

9. **Goals of Oxygen Therapy** 51
   Vikram Damaraju, Inderpaul Sehgal

10. **Drive to Breathe and Carbon Dioxide Retention** 55
    Prashant Nasa, Deven Juneja

11. **Oxygen Transport** 59
    Ujwala Mhatre Ahluwalia, Kapil Borawake

12. **Oxyhemoglobin Dissociation Curve** 64
    Srinivas Samavedam, Shabeer Ahmed Khan

13. **Diffusion of Oxygen and its Applied Physiology** 69
    Srinivas Samavedam, Kiran Raghavendra Asrnanna

14. **Pulse Oximetry: Understanding and Limitations** 73
    Kanwalpreet Sodhi, Manender Kumar

15. **Venous and Arterial Blood Gas Analysis** 80
    Rajesh Pande, Maitree Pandey, Jitin Sharma

Section 3: Oxygen Delivery Systems for the Individual Patients

16. **Oxygen-Delivery Devices** 91
    Tapas Kumar Sahoo, Santanu Bagchi, Rajesh Chandra

17. **Humidification** 99
    Vikram Damaraju, Inderpaul Sehgal

18. **High-Flow Nasal Cannula** 103
    Harjit Dumra, Mansi Dandnaik

19. **Hyperbaric Oxygen Therapy** 109
    Gunjan Chanchalani, Sunil Amin, Kanwalpreet Sodhi

20. **Oxygen Toxicity** 115
    Shrikant Sahasrabudhe, Beena Daniel

Section 4: Oxygen Targets

21. **Effects of Hypoxia and Hypoxemia** 123
    Supradip Ghosh, Sonali Ghosh

22. **How does Oxygen Therapy Work?** 128
    Deepak Govil, Divya Pal

23. **Oxygen Therapy and Targets in Disease Specifics** 134
    Sachin Gupta, Deeksha Singh Tomar

Index *139*

SECTION 1

Basic Facts of Oxygen

- **Industrial and Medical Oxygen Production and Differences**
  Balkrishna Nimavat, Abhijit Deshmukh, Kapil Zirpe

- **Medical Piped Gas Structure, Design, and Safety Systems**
  Prajakta Pote, Kapil Zirpe

- **Medical Compressed Gas Cylinder: Handling and Use**
  Vikas Marwah, Deepu K Peter, Robin Choudhary

- **Cryogenic Liquid Medical Oxygen**
  Shikha Sahi, Apoorva Tiwari, Jeetendra Sharma

- **Oxygen Concentrators**
  Khalid Ismail Khatib, Sameer V Kulkarni, Subhal B Dixit

- **Oxygen Hazards and Safety**
  Deven Juneja, Prashant Nasa, Sahil Kataria

- **Oxygen Audit**
  Rahul Pandit

Industrial and Medical Oxygen Production and Differences

CHAPTER

Balkrishna Nimavat, Abhijit Deshmukh, Kapil Zirpe

INTRODUCTION

Oxygen is considered as crucial element of survival for all human beings. Significance of oxygen store and supply came into much limelight in era of COVID-19 pandemic. How the crisis of oxygen gave rise to global concern during the pandemic is witnessed by all. Along with production, it is also very important about storage and transport of the oxygen. This chapter is to review different methods of production of medical oxygen and key differences between industrial and medical oxygen.

We all know that environmental air contains around 21% of oxygen with major component of nitrogen (78%) and other gases. Till now majority of oxygen production was done by process of air separation in air separation unit (ASU). Oxygen produces by this method considered as highest level of pure form up to 99% and most feasible for medical use. This technique helps the healthcare sector for 75 years to deliver large bulk of oxygen of approximately 5,000 tons/day. This type of method requires large plant works under cryogenic distillation process of steel, petroleum, and chemical industries. But the pandemic has made us brain storm for alternative ways for oxygen productions.

Based on different physical property of gases in air, variety of gas separation methods are used to generate oxygen such as using molecular sieve technology based on different size of molecule, separation of gas based on diffusion, using different adsorption molecule, or separation based on different boiling temperature.

Following are the different methods of oxygen productions:
- Cryogenic ASU (most common)
- Oxygen concentrators (limited to home/domiciliary purpose)
- Pressure swing adsorption (PSA) plant
- Vacuum pressure swing adsorption (VPSA) plant
- Deployable Oxygen Concentration System (DOCS) (emergency situation/war).

CRYOGENIC AIR SEPARATION UNIT

In first step of ASU, air is treated to remove most of impurities like hydrocarbons. This pretreated air then passes through multistage compressor and cooling plant. In the cooling plant, air condenses and water vapors are removed. In next step, air passes through zeolite and silica gel absorbent sieve. This process gives more purity by removing remaining hydrocarbons and carbon dioxide. Then the air passes through cryogenic unit which separate the air component based on cooling point/boiling point. The oxygen being heavy settles to the bottom, separated out while nitrogen and argon condensed on top of vessel. The separated oxygen has around 99.5% purity.

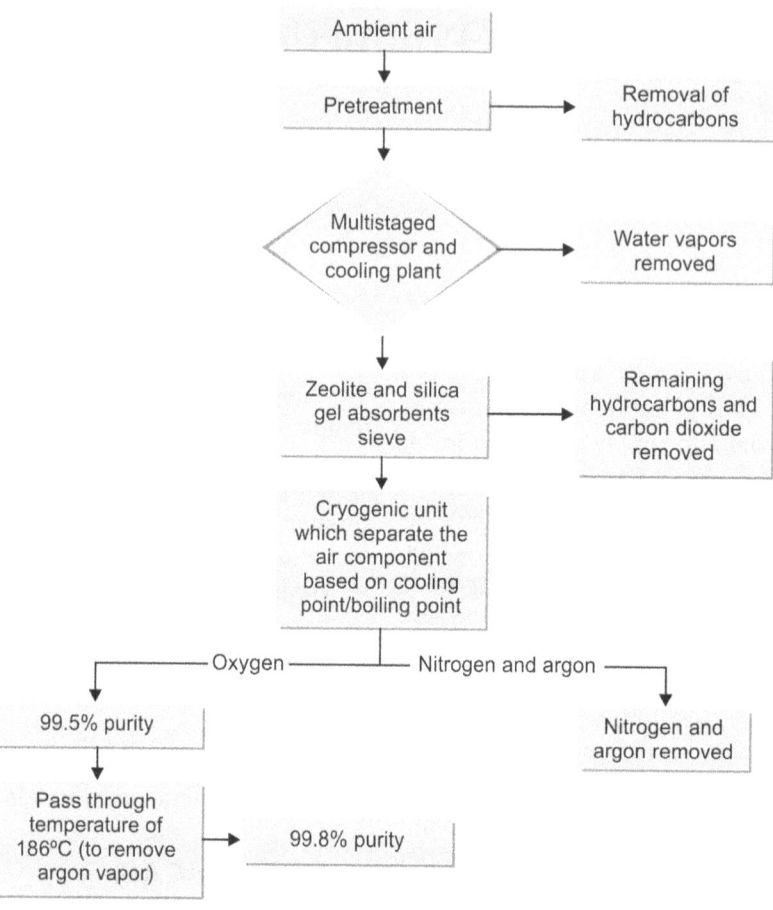

Flowchart 1: Schematic representation of cryogenic air separation unit.

In last phase adding another step of distillation, to achieve 99.8% purity the oxygen has to pass through temperature of 186°C (to remove argon vapor). This type of method requires a large plant, is expensive but is considered best to deliver oxygen in large supply.

PRESSURE SWING ADSORPTION PLANT

Compared to cryogenic ASU, PSA technique use zeolite bed which works as nitrogen adsorbent. Thus, the air coming out is rich in oxygen. PSA does not produce bulk oxygen like cryogenic ASU but it can be alternative or as add-on in case of emergency. They also need constant power supply for generation of oxygen and 1 m^3 generates around 1,000 L of oxygen.

VACUUM PRESSURE SWING ADSORPTION PLANT

This technology was famous in steel or chemical industry for on-site production of oxygen. In this method there is a cyclic swing between overpressure and vacuum that occurs hence the name. The process is similar to PSA except that they use vacuum blower to reduce desorption pressure. Compressed air passes through adsorbent bed where nitrogen, carbon dioxide, and moisture is captured and oxygen-rich air is delivered. Vacuum pump use to desorb the adsorbed nitrogen. Advantages of VPSA over PSA are the use of an oil-free blower thus there is no oil carry-over, the lower operating pressure reduce water condensation allowing better performance in humid environment or high-altitude area. Disadvantage/limitation of this method is— it produces oxygen at purities between 90 and 94%. Most impurities are argon and nitrogen with 4.5 and 5%, respectively.

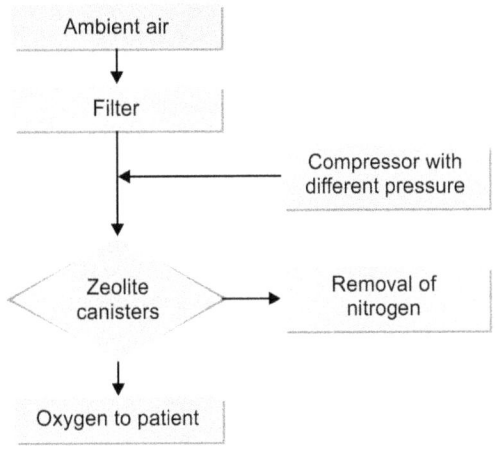

Flowchart 2: Schematic presentation of oxygen concentrator.

DEPLOYABLE OXYGEN CONCENTRATION SYSTEM

This method produces oxygen based on molecular sieve technology and by adsorbing water and nitrogen from filtered air; it is largely used in army or in aerospace division. Deployable oxygen concentration system (DOCS) also are the portable oxygen delivery systems that help in disaster relief situation. It produces oxygen with flow of 30–500 L/min depending on size of unit. It delivers oxygen with 90–96% of purity. Based on Safe Medical Device Act, this type of device is categorized as supplemental and should not be used routinely as life-supporting tool.

OXYGEN CONCENTRATORS

Oxygen concentrators deliver oxygen by compressing the ambient air and removing impurity like nitrogen gas by sieve. Based on level of oxygen concentrators, i.e., home versus commercial they select sieve of ion transport membrane or zeolite material. Main limitations of oxygen concentrators are malfunction of sieve, presence of water vapors affecting nitrogen absorption, persistent supply of room air, and electrical supply. Another pivotal concern is limitation of flow of oxygen as the device generates oxygen of only 0.5–15 L/min depending on low- or high-flow oxygen concentrators. The advantage is— it is portable and feasible for home purpose. As it relies on continuous air supply and electricity cylinder backup is necessary to cover electricity or machine failure.

COMPARISON AMONG VARIOUS OXYGEN PRODUCTION TECHNOLOGIES

Looking at all the options, it is clear that cryogenic ASU is the best option for large volume oxygen in the purest form. In case of crisis, PSA will add-on as rescue measure option for pure form of oxygen. Large volume pure form with PSA is not a cost-effective option compared to cryogenic ASU. Oxygen concentrators are more for home use where requirement of oxygen is not very high **(Table 1)**.

DIFFERENCE BETWEEN MEDICAL OXYGEN AND INDUSTRIAL OXYGEN

Medical oxygen should be standardized by medical grade IP 2010. It is the certificate for oxygen to be used for human. Purity of oxygen

TABLE 1: Comparison among various oxygen production technologies.

	Cryogenic ASU	PSA	Oxygen concentrator
Scale of production	• Large volume production	Intermediate level	• Home purpose • Smaller volume
Purity	Highest level >99%		Up to 95%
Cost	• Costly • Large-area planning	If large scale oxygen by PSA: Not a cost-effective method	Cheaper
Oxygen form	A cryogenic oxygen plant produces both liquid and gaseous oxygen	PSA oxygen plants can only create oxygen in gaseous form	Gas form

(ASU: air separation unit; PSA: pressure swing adsorption)

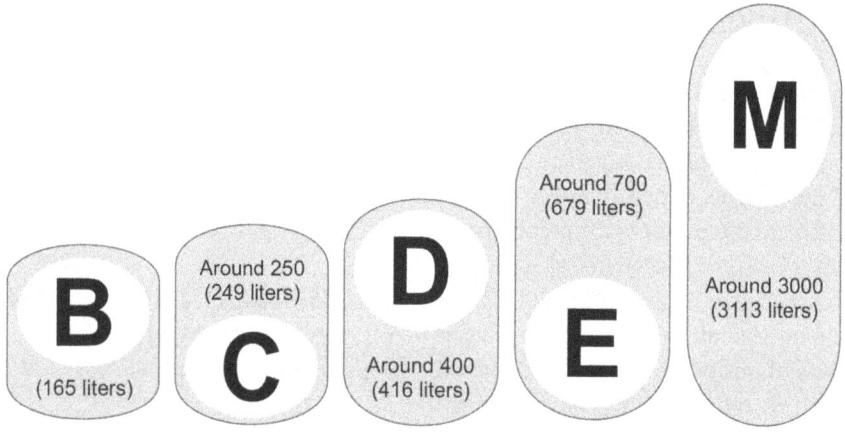

All with serving pressure: 2,015 PSI

Fig. 1: Different oxygen cylinder size and capacity (in brackets values show exact liters in capacity).

should be 99–100%, carbon dioxide level should be ideally <5 ppm, and definitely not >300 ppm, free from halogen, polymer, and moisture and should not cause damage to material like cylinder, gas pipeline, anesthesia machine, or ventilators. It is very important to understand that production of industrial oxygen is not very different than medical oxygen production. However, the difference is in the amount of impurities. Industrial oxygen has higher impurities in the form of other gases, moistures, or carbon dioxide.

DISTRIBUTION AND STORAGE

After production of oxygen at primary plant, oxygen can be transported to secondary plant by two different methods (liquid or gas form) based on capacity of receiving plant. Storage in liquid form is more cost-effective compared to gaseous form. Most of time liquid oxygen (LOX) are stored in insulated double-walled tanks. This tank has outer layer of carbon steel and inner layer of austenitic steel. The outermost layer also has an anticorrosive layer. The space between both layers is filled with insulating powder perlite. Liquid medical oxygen having capacity of around 10,000 L. Gaseous oxygen is stored in cylinders that are made up of steel or aluminium. 1 L of LOX gives 860 L of gaseous oxygen. There are different size cylinders available. Most commonly used in clinical practice are D and E types.

SUGGESTED READING

1. Allam RJ. Improved oxygen production technologies. Energy Procedia. 2008;1:461-70.
2. Jackson M, Shneerson J. An evaluation of the use of concentrators for domiciliary oxygen supply for less than 8 h day-1. Respir Med. 1998;92(2):250-5.
3. Melani AS, Sestini P, Rottoli P. Home oxygen therapy: re-thinking the role of devices. Expert Rev Clin Pharmacol. 2018;11(3): 279-89.
4. Pacific Consolidated Industries. (2007). Expeditionary Deployable Oxygen Concentration System (EDOCS) & mobile oxygen storage tank (MOST). [online] Available from https://www.accessdata.fda.gov/cdrh_docs/pdf6/K061414.pdf [Last accessed June, 2022].
5. Soni NN, Maheshwari DG. Current regulation of medical gases in India and future aspects. Int J Drug Regul Aff. 2018;6(1):35-40.
6. World Health Organization. (2020). Oxygen sources and distribution for COVID-19 treatment centres. [online] Available from https://www.who.int/publications/i/item/oxygen-sources-and-distribution-for-covid-19-treatment-centres [Last accessed June, 2022].

Medical Piped Gas Structure, Design, and Safety Systems

CHAPTER 2

Prajakta Pote, Kapil Zirpe

INTRODUCTION

Gases used for human health care are known as medical gases. These are considered as drugs and are strictly controlled by legislation and standards. Using medical gases by cylinders is inconvenient and costly. Thus medical gas pipeline system (MGPS) has come into existence to provide safe, convenient, and cost-effective way for their delivery. The pipeline system delivers different medical gases, medical air, and provides suction. Area valve service units (AVSUs) are provided for isolating a particular area of the system for service or repair. AVSU comprise of line valves and line valve assemblies. Pressure monitoring and alarm systems are provided for alerting medical staff.

STANDARDS

Different standards have different origins such as ISO 7396-1/2 with origin from European countries, NFPA 99 with USA origin, HTM 2022/0201 with UK origin. There are some similarities and some differences within the different standards (**Table 1**).

COMPONENTS OF A PIPED GAS SYSTEM (FIG. 1)

Manifold

Manifold should be in dedicated room on an outside wall near a loading dock with adequate ventilation. The manifold room should be manned round the clock with trained personnel and should have a suitable acoustic

TABLE 1: Standards of different origins.

ISO 7396	NFPA 99	HTM
All gas sources are triplex plus a maintenance supply assembly	Oxygen sources are duplex or triplex	Oxygen sources are triplex or quadruplex
Vacuum sources are triplex	Vacuum sources are duplex	Vacuum sources are triplex
Multiple receivers are required	Only one receiver is required	Multiple receivers are required
Very limited source sizing guidance given	No source sizing guidance given	Very detailed source sizing guidance
No pipe-sizing guidance given	Sizing minimums are set; no other guidance given	Pipe sizing is detailed in the standard
Location of terminal is not specified	Location of terminal is found in a referenced standard from AIA	Numbers and locations of terminals are specified in the standard

(AIA: American Institute of Architects)

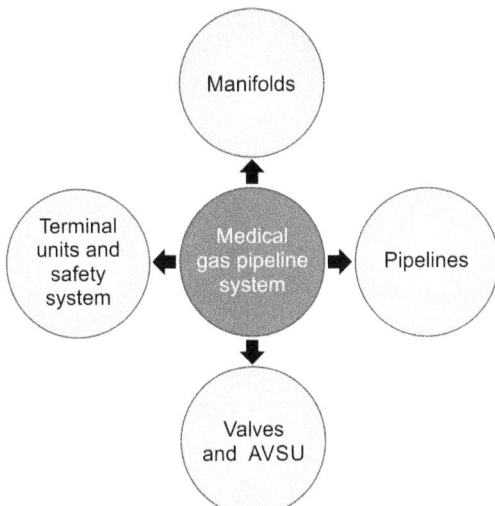

Fig. 1: Components of medical gas pipeline system. (AVSU: area valve service unit)

enclosure along with 100% generator backup and fire security. Cylinder gas or liquid systems should not be in the same room as medical air and compressor vacuum plants. The access to manifold rooms should be from outside and not from corridors or other rooms. At least two doors should be provided to manifold room with one large enough to facilitate handling of cylinders. Internal walls, ceilings and doors should be of a suitable noncombustible 2-hour fire-resistant material as defined in BS 476-4:1970 and BS 476 parts 20–23 (1987). The manifold rooms should not be near high-dependency unit. The location of the manifold rooms should be clearly marked for easy identification in the event of an emergency. The manifold room should have at least two banks of D-type cylinders, each holding a minimum of 2 days consumption, attached to an automatic changeover control panel. As a contingency plan, a 3-day consumption should be kept in reserve at all times.

The pipelines nomenclature are the supply pipeline which are the main hospital pipeline that goes from manifold to building. The feeder pipeline is the horizontal and vertical pipelines that go up to the distribution pipeline. The distribution pipeline is the branch pipeline that serves one floor or a part of it and does not go vertically. And finally the drop pipe is the one from distribution to terminal units.

The pipeline material is a medical grade copper [i.e., phosphorus deoxidized nonarsenical copper confirming to BSEN 1412:1996 grade CW024A (Cu-DHP)]. These copper pipes should have fluxless silver or copper phosphorous brazing as per American Society for Testing and Materials (ASTM) standard and should be intercepted by the AVSUs and alarm panels which display the line pressures and have audiovisual alerts. All pipelines should be color coded with colored bands displayed at every 3 m intervals. Pipes should be seamless, round, solid drawn, suitable for installing vertically or horizontally without sagging or distortion.

Material temper guidelines:
- *For tailpipe:* R220
- *For pipe of 12–54 mm outer diameter:* R250 (half hard)
- *For pipe of outer diameter of >76 mm:* R290 (hard)

All pipelines should be thoroughly checked for any grease, oil, or other combustible material before installation. During brazing of pipe connections (joining two pipes in male to female joint form), the interior of the pipes should be continuously purged with nitrogen. Before installing wall outlets, pipes to be checked for any particulate material. Pressure testing, leaks location, and cross connection testing should be done before installation.

GUIDELINES FOR SUPPORTING MEDICAL GAS PIPELINE SYSTEM PIPELINES (TABLE 2)

Sizing of the Pipes

It is determined by volume of gas to be delivered at what overall pressure. While sizing

TABLE 2: Pipeline support intervals.

Outside diameter (mm)	Maximum intervals	
	For vertical runs (m)	For horizontal runs (m)
12	1.2	1.0
15	1.8	1.2
22–28	2.4	1.8
35–42	3.0	2.4
>54	3.0	2.7

TABLE 4: Color coding of pipelines for different gases.

Gas	ISO standards
Oxygen	White
Nitrous oxide	Blue
Air	Black and white
Vacuum	Yellow
Carbon dioxide	Grey

TABLE 3: Sizing of pipelines.

Operating rooms, pre- and postoperative wards	No pipe smaller than 15 mm OD should be used
Medical vacuum services	No pipe smaller than 15 mm OD should be used

(OD: outside diameter)

for medical vacuum, always provide pipes of one size higher diameter to prevent clogging **(Table 3)**.

Color Coding for Pipelines (Table 4)

Valves and AVSU: All valves are universally of lever-ball type which open and close with 90° rotation. Handle is in line with the pipeline when open **(Fig. 2)**.

Valve positions should be as follows:
- *Main line valve:* Source shut-off valve is provided at outlet of the supply source.
- *Branch valves:* At the base of risers and at every major branch. Placed at secure location.
- *Line valve assembly:* At entry and exit of each section
- *Zone valves:* At each fire zone

All the valve positions should be marked in floor evacuation plan and accessible to floor and for staff.

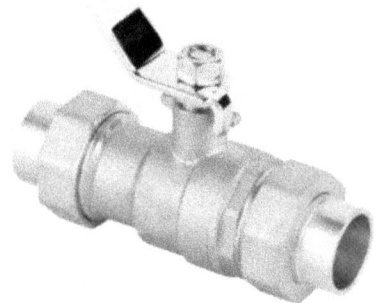

Fig. 2: Lever ball type valve.

Area valve service units (Fig. 3): When the area valves are provided with noninterchangeable screw thread (NIST) gas connectors and gas pressure switch and pressure gauge, it is called AVSU. It can be single or multi gas service units. AVSU are generally installed near the nursing station. AVSU is for isolation of a particular area during servicing in case of gas alarms.

TERMINAL UNITS AND SAFETY SYSTEM (FIG. 4)

There are different terminal units which can be single-gas outlet unit or bed-head panels or trunking system. Bed-head panels along with providing the gas outlets also house nurse call system, flow-meter, infusion pump, reading light, etc. Trunking systems are running panels along the walls similar to bed-head panels.

CHAPTER 2: Medical Piped Gas Structure, Design, and Safety Systems

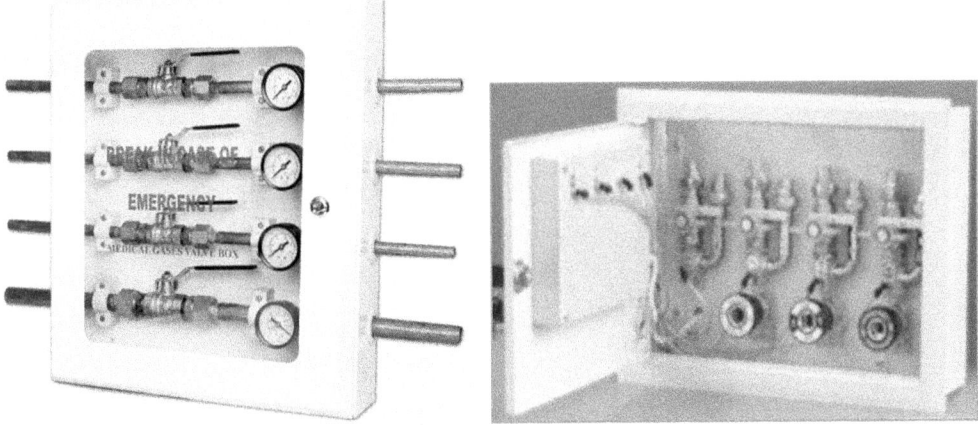

Fig. 3: Area valve service units.

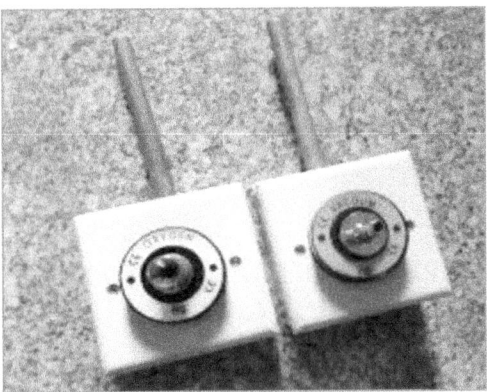

Fig. 4: Terminal units.

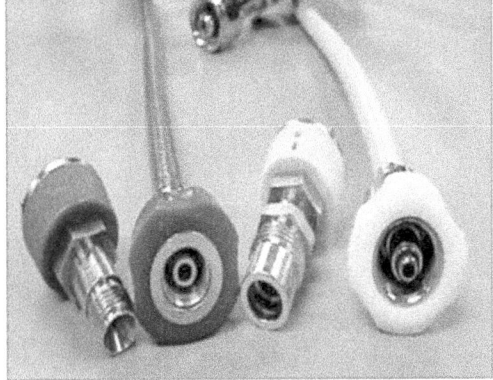

Fig. 5: Diameter Index Safety System.

Terminal units allow plugging of probes from front and has push to insert and press to release mechanism for probes. Self-sealing valves after disengaging of the probe are provided to prevent leaking of gases. They are color coded with gas-specific front plate.

Safety systems: There are different safety systems that are used at terminal units for prevention of wrong connections.

Noninterchangeable screw thread connector: Gas-specific connectors are used at the termination of flexible hoses and copper pipe in MGPS. Dimensions of the male part of the connector make it gas-specific.

Examples are diamond-type oxygen-outlet or chemetron-type oxygen-outlet connectors.

Diameter Index Safety System (DISS): It is a noninterchangeable, threaded fitting to connect gas-powered devices to station outlets (**Fig. 5**).

PIN INDEX SYSTEM

Pin index system is used in small cylinders. It consists of small pins projecting from inner surface of the yoke. They are arranged in such a way that they fit into the corresponding holes in the cylinder valves. The holes are in the arc below the outlet port on the cylinder valve; the

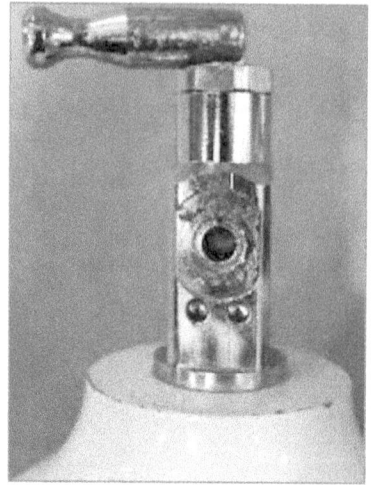

Fig. 6: Pin index on cylinder valve.

Gas	Pin index
Oxygen	2,5
Nitrous oxide	3,5
Carbon dioxide	2,6
Air	1,5
Cyclopropane	3,6
O_2–CO_2 (CO_2 <7.5%)	2,6
O_2–CO_2 (CO_2 >7.5%)	1,6
O_2–He (He >80.5%)	4,6
O_2–He (He <80.5%)	2,4
Entonox	7

TABLE 5: Pin index for particular gases.

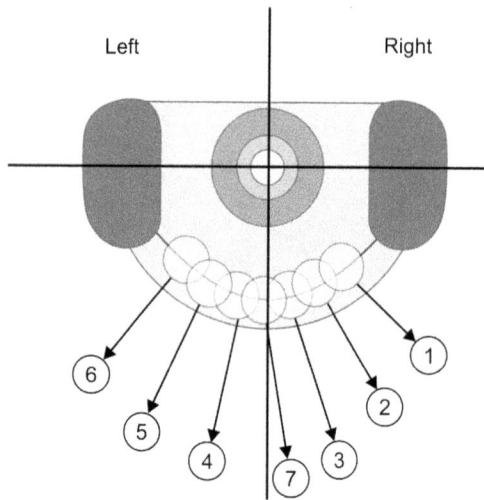

Fig. 7: Pin index system.

port will not seat against the washer of the yoke unless the pins and holes align with each other. There are seven positions of pins and holes and different combinations are fixed for particular gases. Pin index system is also used when the cylinders are being filled so as to avoid wrong gas being filled into the cylinder (**Figs. 6** and **7** and **Table 5**).

Problems with pin index system: If two washers are placed on the port, then the pin index is nullified and a wrong cylinder can be placed on the yoke. If the pins are broken then wrong cylinder can be attached to the yoke.

SPECIFIC DESIGNS FOR SPECIFIC GAS DELIVERY

Oxygen Delivery Systems

Medical oxygen can be >99 or 93%. It can be delivered by individual gas cylinders or gas cylinder manifolds via piping system or through liquid oxygen tank via piping system. 93% medical oxygen is supplied through pressure swing adsorption (PSA) technology via piping system. Oxygen sources comprise of three supplies primary, secondary, and reserve. Piped oxygen is supplied at pressure of 4 bar (400 kPa). A pressure drop of 5% is taken into consideration as allowance. The average oxygen consumption for ward patient is assumed to be 10 L/min/patient and the average oxygen consumption for intensive care unit (ICU) and operative patient is assumed to be 100 L/min/patient.

Oxygen Manifolds

From source to terminal units.

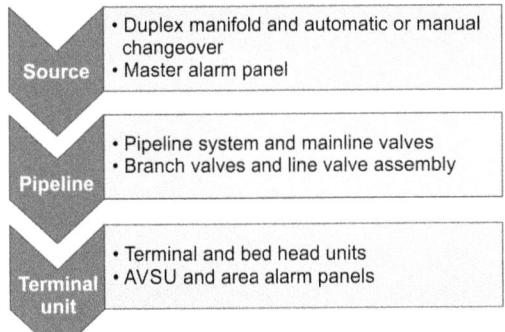

Oxygen manifolds are duplex control manifold with automatic changeover connected to two header bars. It is high pressure low-flow system **(Fig. 8)**. Maximum 10 cylinders are attached in each bank. All cylinders should stand vertically and chained. Each port is connected to cylinder by flexible pigtail connector. The changeover from duty to standby bank is automatic and is based on pneumatic pressure. Master audiovisual alarm is installed at place of manifold technician and is set at 10–20% drop inline pressure.

Liquid medical oxygen is a low pressure high-flow supply system **(Fig. 9)**. The tank is made of stainless-steel inner pressure vessel that is supported in a mild steel outer shell duly insulated in between.

Vacuum System

It is the most commonly used medical gas pipeline services used. Bank of multiple vacuum pumps of small capacity is deployed as

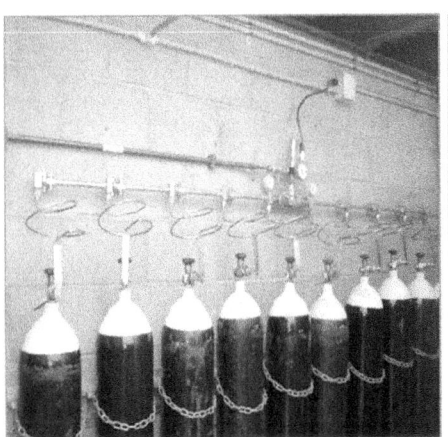
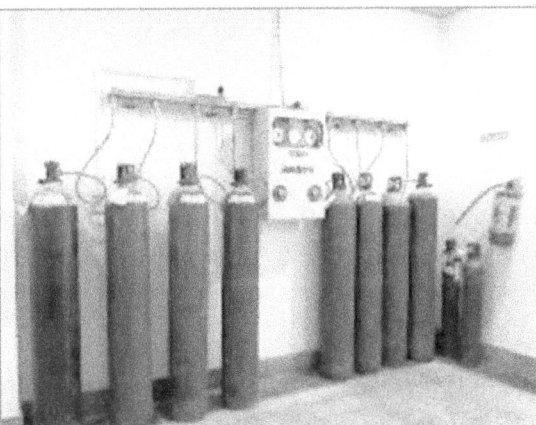
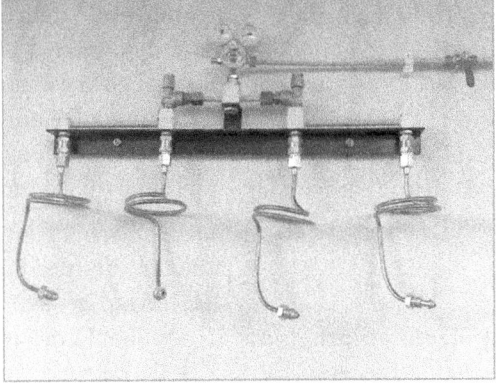

Fig. 8: Oxygen manifold design.

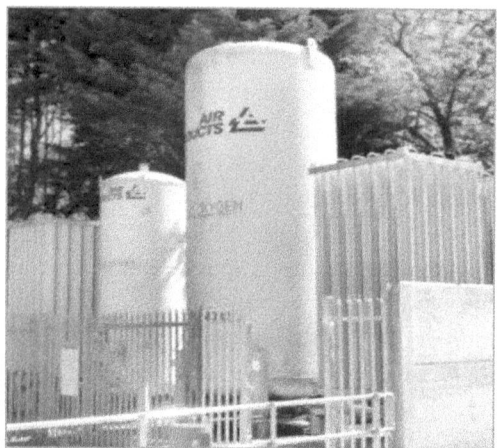

Fig. 9: Liquid medical oxygen tank.

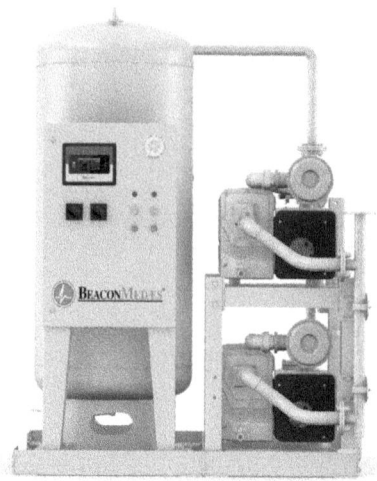

Fig. 10: Duplex vacuum pump.

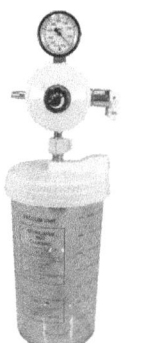
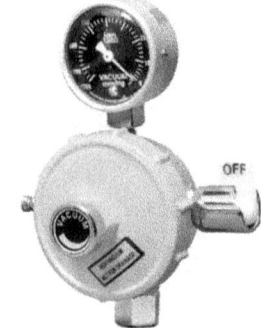

Fig. 11: Ward vacuum unit with regulator.

a multiplex system to use in wards, operation theaters (OTs), ICUs, etc. The suction pressure can be regulated at terminal unit manually by healthcare provider. It is designed to maintain vacuum at 300 mm Hg (40 kPa) at each terminal unit **(Figs. 10 and 11)**.

Vacuum bottles are available in different sizes from 250 mL to 2 L. A suction catheter is connected to the terminal unit.

MEDICAL AIR

It is considered as manufactured drug on site. Compressed air is used in hospitals for functioning of various equipment such as driving pneumatic drills or ventilators, etc. It is also used as blending agent with medical oxygen while delivering to patient. Medical air is delivered at pressure of 4 bar. Flow of medical air is calculated to be 40 and 80 LPM per point for OT and ICU respectively and for surgical use (pneumatic tourniquet or bone saw) almost 350 L/min at 7 bar may be needed.

Components of medical air (Fig. 12): An assembly of three filters are there for delivery of clean air.
1. Prefilter (5 or 1 µm)
2. Fine/bacterial filter (0.01 µm)
3. Coal filter/tower

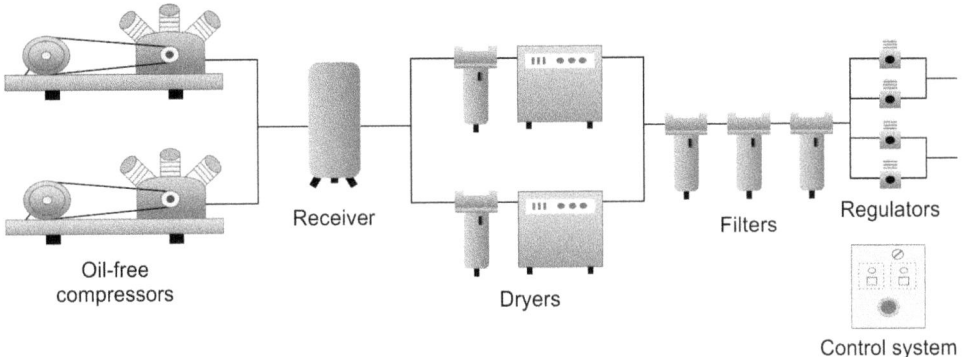

Fig. 12: Components of medical air.

With the help of filter assembly (IS/ISO 7396-1 class) appropriate air quality is achieved. However, the filters have to be checked regularly for clogging.

CONCLUSION

Adequate quality control and safety can be ensured only when there is a proper maintenance of the system. This can be done with various steps such as having 24 hours manning by trained personnel with their periodic training and conducting mock drills of pipeline failure, fire and explosion, formulating standard operating procedures, and maintaining logbooks and finally having preventive maintenance of equipment along with having maintenance contracts from reliable service providers.

SUGGESTED READING

1. Central Public Works Department. Guidelines for medical gas pipeline system. [online] Available from https://www.cpwd.gov.in/images/AzadikaAmrit/MGPS290921.pdf [Last accessed June, 2022].
2. Dorsch JA, Dorsch SE (Ed). Understanding Anesthesia Equipment, 5th edition. Philadelphia: Lippincott Williams and Wilkins; 2007.
3. KG Wentink, RD Jackson (Ed). Medial Gas and Vacuum Systems. Plumbing Systems and Design; 2006. pp. 44-53.
4. Medical vacuum and gas systems. Austin: The University of Texas, MD Anderson Cancer Center; 2010.

Medical Compressed Gas Cylinder: Handling and Use

CHAPTER

Vikas Marwah, Deepu K Peter, Robin Choudhary

INTRODUCTION

Medical gas cylinders have been used for the treatment of millions of patients at healthcare centers and at homes. They comprise oxygen, nitrous oxide, carbon dioxide, air, entonox, and helium. These are compressed and stored in cylinders in liquid or gaseous form. These gases are predominantly used in medical procedures, some for inducing anesthesia and others for driving devices like ventilators, cryoprobe, etc. Improper storage, handling, and use of gas cylinders can pose a physical and chemical threat to both staff and patients. Many patients with diseases like chronic obstructive pulmonary disease with respiratory failure were already on domiciliary oxygen. The recent COVID-19 pandemic left many patients fighting for their lives and in those who survived, the residual pulmonary damage led to increased prescription of domiciliary oxygen therapy.

Reckless use of cylinders is associated with high chances of accidents. We must be aware and also impart knowledge regarding the handling of cylinders to our patients. In this chapter, the basics of medical gas cylinders will be dealt with and we will also learn how to store these cylinders safely at hospitals and home.

COMPONENTS OF A CYLINDER

Medical gas cylinders were previously constructed using steel. Each cylinder has three components: body, shoulder, and neck. The upper part of the body, known as the shoulder, is curved and narrows down to the neck. The neck harbors a screw thread which attaches to the valve. Manufacturers have since moved onto use aluminium, chrome molybdenum steel, or composite materials to make cylinders lighter and can hold a larger volume of gas. Cylinders made of aluminium are considerably lightweight and nonmagnetic and these properties make them ideal for magnetic resonance imaging (MRI) suites and onboard helicopter ambulances. Composite cylinders are made up of lightweight steel or aluminium and encased with Kevlar, Twaron, glass fiber, and polypropylene jacket. These cylinders have the added advantage of being highly durable and can withstand pressures up to 4,000 kPa. Newer cylinders come equipped with flow meters to ensure adequate flow.

To the neck of each cylinder is attached a valve through which gas is filled and discharged. A stem or shaft is connected to each valve. Opening the valve will move the stem upward and closing of valve leads to the stem sealing against the valve thereby moving the gas in and out of the cylinder, respectively. Gas exits from the cylinder through its port. Care should be taken to avoid confusion with the conical depression opposite to the valve as any attempt to screw the retaining screw into the port can cause damage. A packed valve or direct-acting valve is commonly seen in medical gas cylinders and in this system the seat turns when the stem is turned. They can withstand high pressures and prevents leaks through the sealing of the stem with materials like Teflon. The diaphragm valve however has a metal seal and a disk or diaphragm separates the upper and lower stem. These stems may be permanently sealed to the diaphragm. The diaphragm is effective in preventing leakage from the stem. Only a one-half to three-quarter turn can open this valve and since the seat does not turn there is minimal chance of a leak. These properties make it ideal for low pressures and flammable gases.

A cylinder can be opened or closed using a handwheel or handle. Large cylinders usually have a handle attached to it permanently. Smaller cylinders have valve handles of different sizes and shapes. Some handles contain hexagonal opening which can be used to tighten the packing nut. Untrained personnel may use this hexagonal handle, in an attempt to open the valve, might accidentally loosen the packing nut causing the rapid release of compressed gas with force.

The cylinder pressure for oxygen is around 1,800–2,200 psi, for N_2O is 750 psi, and for CO_2 is around 850 psi (5000 kPa). The critical temperature of the gas is the temperature above which a substance cannot be liquefied no matter how much pressure is applied. The critical temperature for oxygen is 118°C and for N_2O is 36.5°C. Gases exists in the gaseous state at room temperature as it is above its critical temperature and hence liquefaction at room temperature cannot occur.

The filling ratio of the cylinder is the weight of the fluid in the cylinder divided by the weight of water required to fill the cylinder.

The service pressure is the maximum pressure up to which the cylinder can be filled at 70°F and testing pressure is usually 1.66 times the working pressure.

Avagadro's law can be used to calculate the quantity of gas in the cylinder. The law states that 1 g molecular weight of any substance will give rise to 22.4 L of gas. The molecular weight of oxygen is 32 and N_2O is 44. Thus the quantity of gas can be calculated by weighing the cylinder to its TARE weight.

TESTING OF CYLINDERS

There are various methods for testing the quality of cylinders such as the Hydraulic test which is the measure of cylinders elasticity. The cylinder is connected by a thread to testing unit, filled with water and the water level is measured by gauge. The gauge is isolated and cylinder pressurized to 240 atmospheres. The pressure is released and the gauge is opened. The cylinder should stretch <0.02%. In the flattening test the cylinder is kept between two compression blocks and pressure is applied from both sides until the distance between blocks remains six times the thickness of the wall of cylinder. The walls should not crack. The tensile test is done in 1 in 100 cylinders and the yield point should not be <15 tons per square inch. In the impact test three longitudinal and three transverse stripes are taken from a finished cylinder and struck by a mechanical hammer. The mean energy to produce the crack should not be <5 and 10 lb/ft for transverse and longitudinal strips, respectively.

PIN INDEX SAFETY SYSTEM

To facilitate the connection of appropriate gas to its valve there is a specific arrangement of pins on each medical gas cylinder. This system is known as the Pin Index Safety System (PISS) and consists of pins protruding from the gas cylinder tank yoke and will fit into appropriate holes in the cylinder valves. The PISS was introduced in 1917, however, its widespread institution did not happen till after World War II wherein a large number of surgeries led to the identification of improvement in the medical gas.

Each cylinder is provided with two pins separated by 12°. The pins are distributed in a semicircular fashion and the first one is located 30° horizontal to the yoke. The pins are designated by numbers depending on their distance in millimeters from the yoke. Over the years there have been numerous changes to improve the quality of PISS. This system should not be considered foolproof and the staff should always be vigilant while monitoring the gas delivery during anesthesia.

IDENTIFICATION OF CYLINDERS

Different compositions of gases and their combination are used for medical purposes. To ensure that the correct gas is administered safely and to prevent any confusion color coding has been prescribed. The color coding followed in our country is being depicted in **Table 1**. The color on each cylinder can vary depending on the paint used and there can be variations in color tone. Also, the color perceived by each user might be different. Hence color alone should not be used for identification and the identity should be confirmed with the label before putting a cylinder to use. Color alone should be identified only for arranging and sorting the cylinders.

Cylinders come in various sizes and each size is designated a letter based on the capacity. The sizes of commonly used cylinders are given in **Table 2**. Size ranges from 1.2 to 6,550 L. Size E cylinders are most commonly used on anesthesia machines.

STORAGE

All medical gas cylinders should be stored in a dry, cool, and clean area which has been designated as "storage area". This area should be away from the operating room and should be adequately ventilated and covered and away from boilers, open flames, steam pipes, and any source of heat and fire. As most gas cylinders are prone to catch fire easily, storage area should be made of fire-resistant

TABLE 1: Color coding used for identification of medical gas cylinders.

Name of gas	Color
Air	White and black
Carbon dioxide	Grey
Cyclopropane	Orange
Ethylene	Violet
Helium	Brown
Mixture of oxygen and carbon dioxide	White and grey
Mixture of oxygen and helium	White and brown
Nitrogen	Black
Nitrous oxide	Blue
Oxygen	White

Source: Srivastava U. Anaesthesia gas supply: gas cylinders. Indian J Anaesth. 2013;57(5):500-6.

TABLE 2: Various sizes of oxygen gas cylinders available.

Size	Capacity (L)	Pressure (psi)	Tare weight (kg)	Valve type
B	200	1,900	2.27	Pin
D	400	1,900	3.4	Pin
E	660	1,900	5.4	Pin
F	1,360	1,900	14.5	Bull nose
G	3,400	1,900	34.5	Bull nose
H	6,900	2,200	53.2	Bull nose
M	3,450	2,200	29	Bull nose

Source: Srivastava U. Anaesthesia gas supply: gas cylinders. Indian J Anaesth. 2013;57(5):500-6.

materials and the wrappings on each cylinder should be removed prior to storing.

To prevent tampering with these cylinders, the storage areas should be accessible to only authorized trained personnel. Public access to these areas should not be allowed and smoking should be completely prohibited in premises where cylinders are stored. Cylinders should not be draped with any material as combustible materials can accumulate under the drape and can lead to a fire. Cylinders especially nitrous oxide and oxygen being highly flammable should be stored away from combustible materials. If the storage area is in the open, it should be ensured that the cylinders are not exposed to extreme heat and cold weather and the temperature of the cylinder should not go beyond 125° or below 10°.

They should not be stored in a place wherein they can become part of an electric arc and can get damaged. Care should be taken to not subject the cylinders to mechanical shock and the storage area should have a flat and strong base.

Cylinders should be arranged in such a way that the earlier supplied cylinders should be used first and the proper segregation of full and empty cylinders are done to prevent unwanted delays during an emergency. The personnel in charge should also maintain a complete inventory of the cylinders and the grouping of cylinders is also done as per content, size, and color.

HANDLING AND INSTALLATION

Each gas cylinder should be identified using its color coding and label. In case of a missing or illegible label, the cylinder should be returned to the manufacturer. Only authorized and trained personnel who understand the potential hazards should be allowed to handle cylinders. Even an unserviceable cylinder should be handled by personnel qualified to dispose off the same.

Any damage to a cylinder can pose a safety hazard and the supplier/owner should be informed about the damage. It has to be emphasized that most individuals involved in the transport and storage of cylinders are not aware of safe handling practices. Care should be taken not to drag, roll, slide or drop the cylinder or fall upon one another and that the valve is not used for lifting or moving the cylinder.

Repainting, tampering, alteration or the repair of the cylinder, pressure-relief devices, and valve should be done only by trained individuals. The valve is usually wrapped with a tamper-evident seal which has to be removed before use.

The valve cover cap of bull-nose cylinders should be retained for attachment after use. The valve should be turned off and closed except when being used. Oil, grease, and other lubricants should not be used especially in the valves, regulators, or gauges as they are easily combustible.

Excess force should not be applied while opening valves or attaching connectors. The appropriate cylinder key should be used for opening and the valve should be turned anticlockwise to its full extent followed by a quarter turn clockwise. Hammering of the valve should be avoided. While being used the valve has to be fully opened to prevent faulty delivery of the gas.

Ensure that there are no leaks by listening or by using leak detection fluid. Attempts can be made to remedy the leak by replacing the washer or by screwing the packing nut in a clockwise manner without undue force. If any leak which cannot be corrected by tightening the connections is present, the cylinder should be closed, removed from the manifold, and returned to the supplier with a faulty label attached to it. Any unexpected loss in pressure, despite not using the cylinder, should warrant evaluation for a slow leak.

Prior to attaching a cylinder to a machine, the regulator should also be inspected for any damages, and foreign particles. A pressure regulator ensures that the pressure of the released gas is at usable levels and can prevent accidents arising out of gas release at high pressures. Turning the valve slowly allows to prevent the rapid filling of gas in the space between the valve and yoke and thereby allowing more time for heat dissipation. If any particles of dust and grease are present in this space, rapid filling of gas can lead to fire.

After the valve is opened, the pressure has to be checked again and cylinders with very high pressure, much more than anticipated, should be returned to the supplier.

After usage, the valve has to be completely closed and the valve cap placed back. An empty cylinder should be labeled as "EMPTY" and closing the valve will prevent leakage of any leftover gas.

Dangers of Improper Handling and Storage

Despite numerous safety measures like color coding and PISS, safety hazards related to medical gas cylinders are still reported. Excessive and repeated use leads to fading of the color coding and thereby wrong identification. Color coding on a particular cylinder can itself be incorrect. Also there have been instances where a wrong gas was filled or a wrong label was attached on the cylinder. Pins on the cylinder can be broken due to poor maintenance. This can result in attachment of wrong cylinder to a regulator or yoke. Cases have also been reported in which wrong gases were administered during surgeries due to incorrectly filled cylinders.

The valve can be damaged and release its contents if the screw is incorrectly screwed into the safety relief device. Rapid release of contents of a cylinder especially nitrous oxide into a confined oxygen deficient room can result in asphyxia and death.

Cylinder fires and explosions were seen when oxygen equipment was contaminated with oil, grease, paraffin, or dirt. Overfilling of cylinders was also identified as one of the causes of explosion of gas cylinders. Placing a cylinder with a jerk on a hard surface can cause mechanical shock and an explosion. There has been instances where individuals lifted the cylinder while holding the valve which might have led to leakage of gas and placing the same cylinder on the ground with a jerk resulted in an explosion.

Non-MR compatible cylinders have accidentally become projectiles and have caused injuries to individuals and damage to the MRI machine.

If a cylinder falls and the valve breaks the pressurized gas can rapidly escape and the cylinder can become a projectile rocket and spin out of control and lead to damage to people and property.

LIQUID OXYGEN

The COVID pandemic caused widespread loss to human life, and many were left with residual lung disease and had to be placed on domiciliary oxygen. Liquid oxygen is small and compact, and was kept in many households during the pandemic. It is also used while transferring patients and for emergency use by mountaineers. While handling and storing liquid oxygen cylinders all precautions as mentioned earlier should be taken.

Spills from liquid oxygen can happen during accidents while carrying these portable cylinders. The oxygen from the spill should be given time to dissipate and no contact with the skin should be made as any contact with the liquid oxygen or the valves with liquid oxygen frosting can cause burns.

As seen with other gas cylinders, these cylinders should also be kept free from combustible materials like oils, grease, and foreign particles. These can lead to fires and any further spill can increase the chance of the spread of the fire. These cylinders should also not be subjected to extremes of temperature and physical damage while handling should be avoided.

CONCLUSION

Medical gas cylinders are used extensively in both hospitals and at homes. They contain gases in liquid or gaseous form and harbor numerous inbuilt safety features. Personnel should be regularly trained about the proper use of gas cylinders and the hazards involved and only trained personnel should be allowed to handle them. Identification of the cylinders through their labels and color coding will prevent operation room accidents. Our knowledge of storage, handling, and use of medical gas cylinders will help prevent accidents related to cylinders, can help deliver proper health care to patients and will help create a safe environment to work.

SUGGESTED READING

1. Colletti PM. Size "H" oxygen cylinder: accidental MR projectile at 1.5 Tesla. J Magn Reson Imaging. 2004;19(1):141-3.
2. Crombie N. Confusing and ambiguous labelling of an oxygen cylinder. Anaesthesia. 2009;64(1):98-98.
3. Gupta S, Jani CB. Oxygen cylinders: "life" or "death"? Afr Health Sci. 2009;9(1):57-60.
4. Hogg CE. Pin-indexing failures. Anesthesiology. 1973;38(1):85-7.
5. Medical gas safety. Read the labels! They're the only sure identifier of gas cylinder contents. Health Devices. 2001;30(3):87-9.
6. Menon MRB, Lett Z. Incorrectly filled cylinders. Anaesthesia. 1991;46(2):155-6.
7. Obeidat A, Andreas T, Bordas SPA, Zilian A. Simulation of gas-dynamic, pressure surges and adiabatic compression phenomena in geometrically complex respirator oxygen valves. Therm Sci Eng Prog. 2021;24.
8. Srivastava U. Anaesthesia gas supply: gas cylinders. Indian J Anaesth. 2013;57(5):500-6.
9. Tracey JA, Kennedy J, Magner J. Explosion of carbon dioxide cylinder. Anaesthesia. 1984;39(9):938-9.

Cryogenic Liquid Medical Oxygen

CHAPTER

Shikha Sahi, Apoorva Tiwari, Jeetendra Sharma

INTRODUCTION

Oxygen, synonymous with "the Dephlogisticated Air" of Joseph Priestley, is one of the most important prerequisite conditions for existence of life on earth. Amusingly, it was in fact the two most vital capabilities of this component of air, the ability to support combustion ("a candle would burn") and respiration ("a mouse would thrive"), which led to the discovery of oxygen. Oxygen therapy is the administration of oxygen at concentrations greater than ambient air, with the intent of treating the symptoms and manifestations of hypoxia with applications both at hospital and at home. As per Indian Pharmacopoeia's specifications, medical grade oxygen (IP 2010) should have 99.0–100% purity; does not damage gas cylinders, pipelines, anesthesia machines, or ventilators; and hence certified safe for human use. It should also be free from halogen, polymer, oxidizing substances, and moisture with particulate count of carbon monoxide and carbon dioxide <5 parts per million (ppm) and 300 ppm, respectively. Albeit, the World Health Organization (WHO) states that medical oxygen should be at least 82% pure, free from any contamination, and produced by oil-free compressor.

OXYGEN DELIVERY EQUIPMENT

Hospitals rely largely on large liquid oxygen (LOX) storage tanks as their primary oxygen source distributed to the bedside by medical gas pipeline system (MGPS). It is safer, less cumbersome, and cost-effective than compressed gas cylinders which are primarily reserved for patient transport and backup in case of MGPS failure. The oxygen source for home oxygen therapy can be oxygen concentrators, compressed gas cylinders, or LOX, all three being available in stationary and portable versions. Due to characteristics peculiar to every oxygen source and wide variability in oxygen needs of patients attributable to underlying lung disease, activity level, and oxygen flow requirements, careful prescription of the oxygen source at the start of home oxygen therapy is critical in meeting patient demands, ensuring patient adherence and improving quality of life.

CRYOGENIC LIQUID MEDICAL OXYGEN

Cryogenic liquids are liquefied gases with boiling point below –130°F (–90°C). Oxygen liquefies at a temperature of –183°C into pale blue and extremely cold liquid called cryogenic LOX. LOX solidifies at a temperature of –218°C. Oxygen is liquefied primarily for the storage advantage and it must be vaporized to a gas state prior to use. Vaporization of 1 L of LOX produces 860 L of gaseous oxygen. This expansion ratio of 860:1 allows large quantities of oxygen (gas) to be stored as a liquid (LOX) in a small receptacle making LOX the most efficient system for oxygen storage and transportation.

MANUFACTURE

Oxygen can be produced both cryogenically and noncryogenically. Cryogenically produced LOX is always generated offsite in bulk quantities in air separation units (ASUs) by the air separation and cryogenic distillation process. Dr Carl von Linde invented the technique of double column rectification system and cryogenic air separation in 1910, making it possible to produce pure oxygen and pure nitrogen simultaneously.

Liquid Oxygen Plant (Fig. 1)

Pure gases are separated from air by first cooling it until it liquefies, then selectively distilling the components at their various boiling temperatures. Air is sucked in and filtered to remove gross impurities like heavy hydrocarbons and dust. The filtered air is then compressed to a pressure of 6 bar which condenses and removes water vapors. From here, the air passes through a molecular sieve made of zeolite and silica gel-type absorbents, which trap the remaining carbon dioxide, water vapors, and hydrocarbons which would freeze and plug the cryogenic equipment. The compressed air is cooled to a temperature of –180°C in the heat exchanger and fed into the bottom of Linde double distillation column. As it expands in the separation columns, it cools down still further (reversed bicycle pump effect) and liquefies to some extent (the temperature being lower than the boiling point).

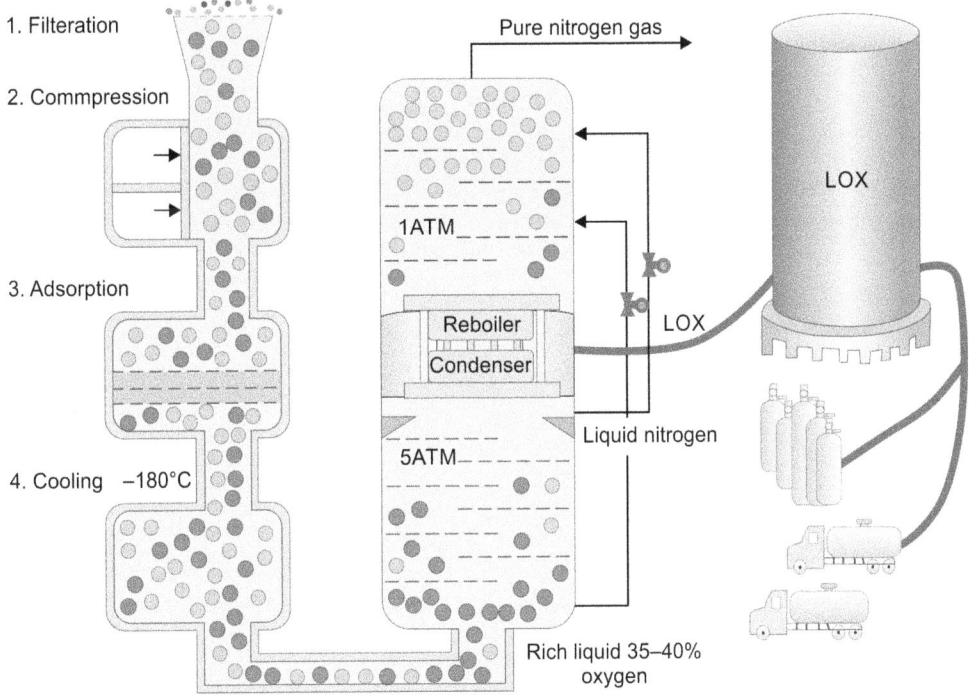

Fig. 1: Cryogenic production of liquid oxygen in an air separation unit based on Linde double column rectification and cryogenic fractional distillation method. (LOX: liquid oxygen)

Linde double column comprises a lower high-pressure column with a condenser at the top and the upper low-pressure column with a reboiler at the bottom. The condenser in the lower column acts as a reboiler for the upper column, the two being thermodynamically coupled. Air separation is a purely physical process, with oxygen (boiling point of −183°C), condensing down to the bottom of the lower column whereas nitrogen (boiling point of −196°C) remaining in the gaseous state. Since argon has a boiling point similar to that of oxygen (−186°C), significant amount of argon liquefies along with oxygen. "Rich liquid" containing 35–40% oxygen, is taken out from the bottom and fed to the center part of the upper column for further separation. The upper column separates pure liquefied oxygen at the bottom and pure nitrogen gas to the top. This technique is designed for high volume production of oxygen (approximately 5,000 tons/day).

CRYOGENIC CONTAINERS

Consequential to the large temperature gradient between the LOX and the surroundings, special equipment is required for handling and storage.

Liquid Medical Oxygen Storage Tanks (Fig. 2)

Liquid medical oxygen (LMO) tanks are the chief and the most common source of oxygen in healthcare facilities. The main LMO tank supplies the centrally piped system (MGPS) throughout the hospital by self-vaporization for which no power supply is required. A typical storage system also called vacuum-insulated evaporator (VIE), consists of a LMO tank, vaporizer, and a pressure control system. LMO tanks are large cylindrical tanks, which are double-walled and vacuum-insulated, with a capacity of 990–10,000 L.

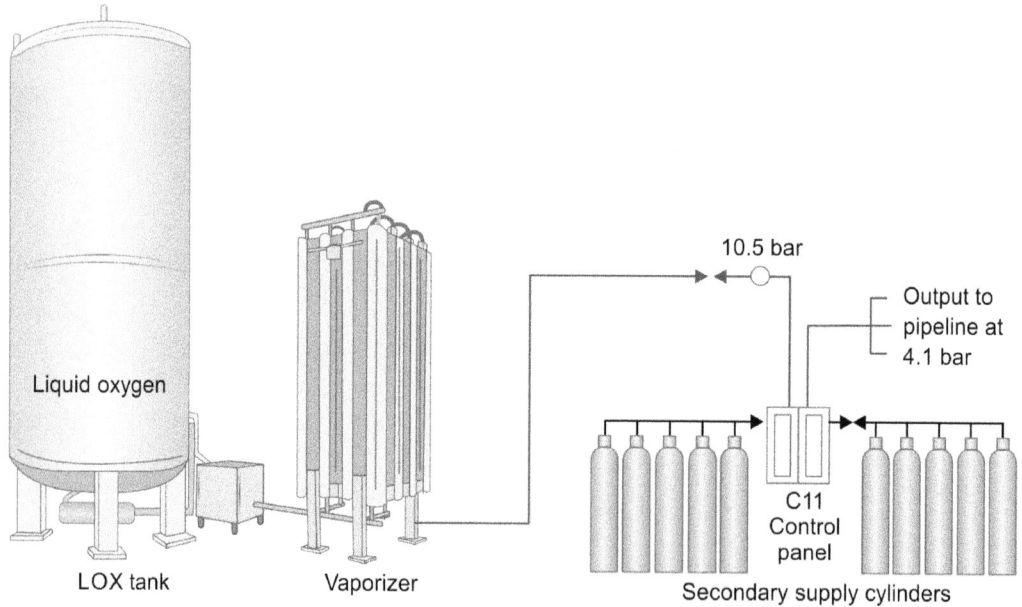

Fig. 2: A typical vacuum-insulated evaporator consists of a liquid medical oxygen tank, vaporizer, and a pressure control system. (LOX: liquid oxygen)

The inner wall is made of stainless steel and the outer wall is made of carbon steel and the space between the two has vacuum or highly insulating perlite. The inner vessel is maintained at pressure near 10.5 bar. An external ambient heated vaporizer allows LOX to be vaporized to the ambient temperature before being supplied to the pipeline system at the working pressure of approximately 4 bar. According to the current regulations for medical gases in India, LMO tanks should be constructed at ground level and in open and unhindered space for the smooth movement of the supply tanker. Natural evaporation rate is maintained to <1%. Low liquid level alarm and backup source of oxygen is mandatory and is usually the D type cylinders attached to the gas manifold. Display of LOX level and outlet pressure is necessary.

Cryogenic Liquid Cylinders

Cryogenic liquid cylinders are pressurized vessels with capacity of 80–450 L. They are pressurized to 350 psig (24 atm) and are equipped with pressure relief valve and rupture disks as safety mechanism. Oxygen may be withdrawn as a gas by passing liquid through an internal vaporizer or as a liquid under its own vapor pressure.

Portable Liquid Oxygen Dewar

A Dewar is named after Scottish Chemist and Physicist James Dewar who invented the vacuum flask. A Dewar is a specialized, double-layered vacuum-insulated flask, intended to thermally insulate the liquid cryogen in order to reduce the rate at which it boils away. Although Dewars are well-insulated and nonpressurized vessels, some heat leak to the interior is unavoidable due to the large temperature gradient. Consequently, the vapors produced collect in the space above the liquid and if not used build pressure (head pressure) inside the vessel. The head pressure is periodically vented via the pressure relief valve as a safety feature of the container. Vaporization rates vary from 0.4 to 3% of the container's volume per day.

Stationary Unit

Dewars are available in different sizes and capacities. The mother unit **(Fig. 3A)** is a large capacity, stationary container installed in the patient's home. Besides providing the storage reservoir for periodically refilling the portable dewars, they are used for continuous flow oxygen therapy in nonambulatory patients. **Figure 3B** illustrates the components of the mother unit. The contents indicator with LED lights at the top indicate the level of LOX in the reservoir. It has a portable fill connector to fill the portable Dewar and a release button to release the portable Dewar after filling. Diameter index safety system (DISS) connector of the reservoir allows attachment of external flow control valve (EFCV), humidifier bottle, tubing adaptor, and nasal cannula in this sequence when breathing directly from the reservoir. Other controls are vent valve, pressure gauge, and a pull out type moisture container.

Portable Unit

Portable dewars are available in 300–600 L gaseous equivalent capacity. Owing to their compact and light weight design, they can be easily carried by the top handle, shoulder strap, or inside the backpack. This maintains the patient's freedom to travel and compliance to the treatment. Components of the potable unit **(Fig. 4)** include carrying handle at the top, flow control knob in the front, fill connector at the bottom, contents indicator strap, contents indicator window, and vent valve lever at the back. Breathing

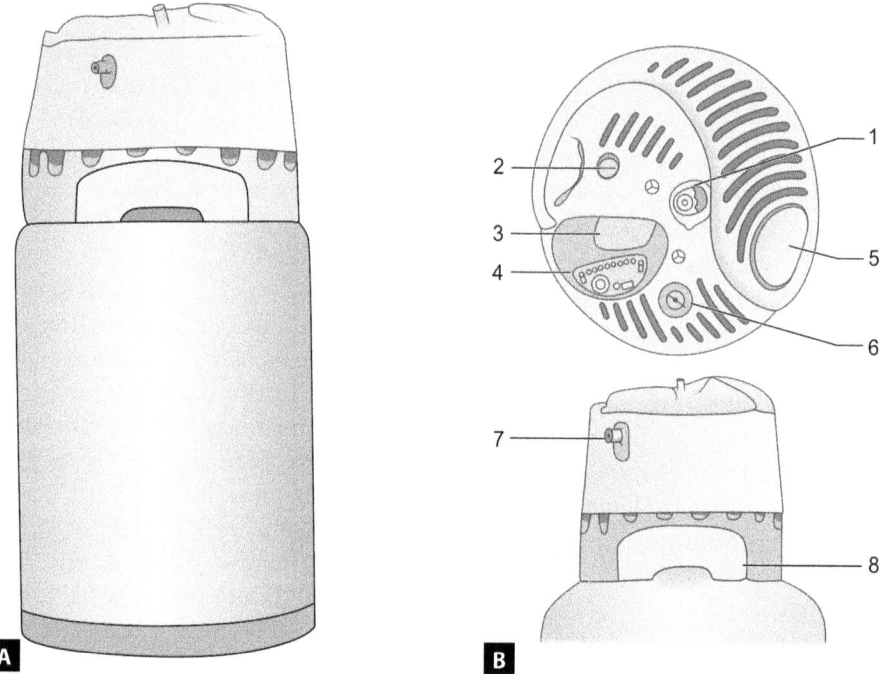

Figs. 3A and B: (A) A stationary unit; (B) The components of the stationary unit: (1) portable fill connector, (2) vent valve, (3) battery housing, (4) contents indicator, (5) portable release button, (6) pressure gauge, (7) diameter index safety system connection (breathing oxygen supply), and (8) moisture container.

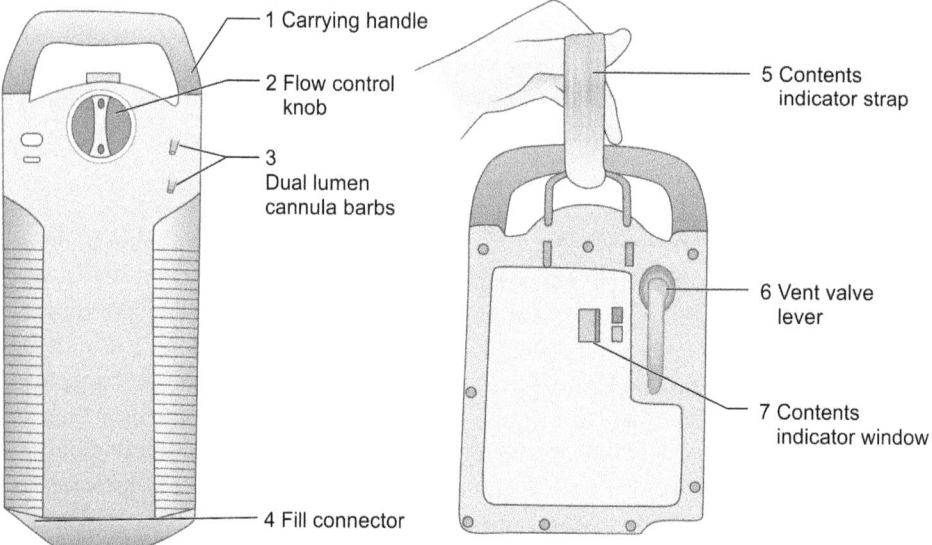

Fig. 4: The components of the portable Dewar: (1) carrying handle, (2) flow control knob, (3) dual lumen cannula barbs, (4) fill connector, (5) contents indicator strap, (6) vent valve lever, and (7) contents indicator window.

CHAPTER 4: Cryogenic Liquid Medical Oxygen

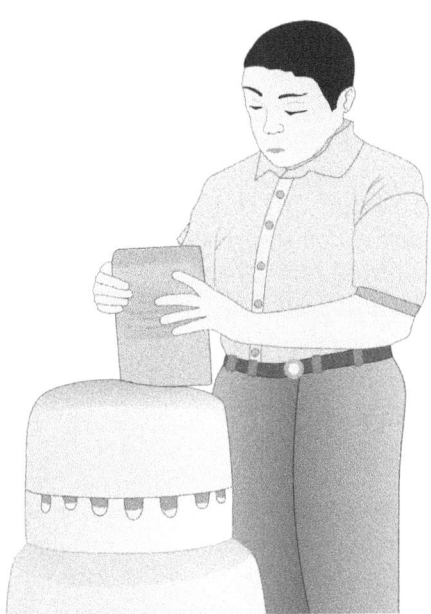

Fig. 5: The filling of the portable unit from the mother unit.

through the portable Dewar requires a double lumen nasal cannula with two connections for the oxygen outlet and sense connector. The beginning of inspiration is sensed at the sense connector allowing oxygen flow only during inspiration. The intermittent flow delivery improves oxygen conservation and time to next refilling.

Portable dewars come in side-fill and top-fill configurations bestowing the patient control over refilling of portable unit from the mother unit. Steps for refilling of portable dewars **(Fig. 5)** include turning the flow control valve to OFF position, cleaning the fill connectors with dry cotton cloth to remove any grease, engaging the portable fill connector with the reservoir fill connector, maintain a constant downward force, pull the vent valve on the portable unit to start the filling which takes 20–30 seconds and produces a hissing sound and some vapors. The vent valve is then released and the portable unit is separated by pushing the release button the reservoir.

HAZARDS AND SAFETY PRECAUTIONS

The potential hazards stem from two properties unique to cryogenic liquids: extremely cold temperature and the expansion ratio. Cryogenic liquids can rapidly freeze human tissue causing frost bite. High-expansion ratio produces an oxygen-enriched atmosphere when LOX is released. Although oxygen itself is nonflammable, combustible materials burn easily and more vigorously. Materials that normally do not burn in air may burn in an oxygen-enriched atmosphere. Following safety precautions should be adhered to while handling cryogenic oxygen containers.

Liquid Oxygen Dewars

- Do not cover vessels. These units normally vent oxygen.
- Keep vessels in upright position. Overturning could result in spillage.
- In case of accidental tip over, cautiously return the unit to upright position. If LOX is escaping, open the windows and leave the area. Do not attempt to move the unit or stop the LOX from escaping.
- Leather or insulated gloves and other protective clothing (long-cuffless pants, long-sleeved shirt, safety glasses, and full face shield) should be worn when operating valves or before touching cold piping.
- Store liquid containers in well-ventilated area.
- Smoking, candles, and open flames are prohibited within 10 feet of the device.
- Vessel valves and associated equipment must never be lubricated and kept free of oils or grease.
- Avoid oil-based creams and petroleum jelly on the face and hands while handling LOX.
- Ensure that all alcohol-based hand rub has evaporated before handling LOX equipment.

Liquid Oxygen Storage Tanks

- No overhead power wires should be constructed over LOX tanks.
- Do not plug, remove, or tamper with any pressure relief device of LOX tanks.
- There should be at least 5 meter vacant space with fencing around the LMO tank.

Liquid Oxygen Cylinders

- LOX cylinders should not be rolled over.
- Transport with a handcart by pushing and not pulling.

BENEFITS OF LIQUID OXYGEN

- Maximum purity of oxygen >99.5%.
- Storage and transport benefits attributable to high-expansion ratio.
- Self-refill at home by patient from stationary containers.
- High flows up to 15 L/min oxygen
- Both continuous and pulse flow options
- *Light weight:* 2.5 kg–4 kg
- Maximum portability allowing long trips away from home
- No batteries or electricity required.
- Easy to operate and filling operations.
- Does not emit heat or noise.
- Low maintenance
- Improves patient adherence.
- Improved health-related quality of life (HRQL).

LIMITATIONS OF LIQUID OXYGEN

- Icing can occur on the heat exchange coils due to the freezing of water vapor of the ambient air. Patients using high-flow LOX usually require two systems, to allow one system to deice while the other is in use.
- Finite capacity necessitating a backup supply.
- *Cost:* Compared to oxygen concentrators, LOX therapy is four times more expensive due to higher equipment acquisition costs and high delivery cost associated with refilling. A base unit with 85 lb LOX capacity when used @2 L/min in demand mode will need refilling after 10 days.
- Difficulty to refill and follow safety instructions especially by elderly patients with cognitive dysfunction.
- Limited availability
- Supplier dependency

USES

Medical

Medical grade oxygen including LOX is used in healthcare settings for management of hypoxemia in acute cardiopulmonary illness [acute respiratory distress syndrome (ARDS), pneumonia, pulmonary edema, pneumothorax, atelectasis, pulmonary embolism], during anesthesia, carbon monoxide poisoning, chest trauma, and hyperbaric oxygen therapy. Domiciliary oxygen therapy involves delivery of oxygen therapy at home in chronically hypoxemic patients. Depending upon the indication and duration therapy, domiciliary oxygen therapy can be long-term oxygen therapy (LTOT), short-term, nocturnal, ambulatory, or palliative therapy. **Table 1** shows comparison between various oxygen sources for home oxygen therapy.

Industrial

Liquid oxygen is manufactured at large scale for industrial use. Albeit the manufacture of industrial oxygen (cryogenic fractional distillation method) is not different from that of the medical oxygen, industrial oxygen may have a comparatively higher percentage of impurities (other gases or particulate impurities), whereas medical oxygen is in its purest form. LOX is widely used as an oxidant

TABLE 1: Comparison between various oxygen sources.

	Pressurized oxygen cylinder	Oxygen concentrator	LOX
Manufacture process	A metal container filled with compressed gaseous oxygen under high pressure (2015 psi service pressure)	A self-contained, electrical device that draws room air into series of filters and molecular sieve which absorb nitrogen to produce concentrated oxygen	LOX is produced in oxygen plants called ASUs via cryogenic fractional distillation process
Oxygen purity	>99%	87–95%	Purest (99% and above)
Flows	Allows delivery of continuous flow oxygen up to 15 L/min	0.5–5 L/min in typical concentrator. Stationary models provide high flows (>10 L/min)	Allows delivery of continuous flow oxygen up to 15 L/min
Size and weight	• Available in multiple sizes from 2.5 to 9 kg • Portable (B, C, D, E, M type) • Fixed (H, K type)	Vary in weight (1.5–10 kg)	Medium to large portable dewars between 2.5 and 4 kg
Refill	Only possible in small cylinders via stationary concentrators, but last <1 hour on continuous-flow rates >3 L/min	Refill is not required. Can supply unlimited amount of oxygen as long as power is available	Patient refills portable canisters from a larger home reservoir of LOX
Electricity requirement	No	Yes, continuously	No
Availability	Easy	Easy	Limited
Use time @2 L/day	2.5 days	Continuous	8.9 days, special system >30 days
Procurement cost	• Low • No installation needed	• Moderate • Easy to install at home	• Four times higher cost • Requires high technical support
Running cost	*High:* Frequent refilling, transport, and logistics	*Small:* Power use, need to change filters	High
Noise	Minimal	Noisy and vibration	Minimal
Patient mobility	Least supportive	Not supportive	Best for ambulatory patients and improves patient mobility
Travel	Not allowed for air travel	POC are the only portable oxygen source allowed for air travel	Not allowed for air travel
User care	Minimal (pressure checks, minimize fire hazards)	Moderate (filter cleaning and device exterior, minimize fire hazards)	Minimal

Contd…

Contd...

	Pressurized oxygen cylinder	Oxygen concentrator	LOX
Advantage	Fulfills all oxygen needs (high-pressure supply, high flows), power independent, provides backup for portable devices	Self-contained (no refill), output flow can be split into multiple patients, easy installation, suitable for air travel	Maximum purity oxygen. Fulfills all oxygen needs (high-pressure supply, high flows), power independent, ambulation, occupy least space, and weight
Disadvantage	Heavy, distributor required, need for accessories (pressure gauge, regulator, flowmeter), explosion, and fire hazard	Power dependent, variable oxygen purity, weight, noise, loss of efficacy at high-flow rate, and tachypnea	Distributor required, frost burns, icing on the equipment, exhaustive supply, high cost, backup cylinder required, fires

(ASU: air separation units; LOX: liquid oxygen; POC: portable oxygen concentrator)

for liquid fuels in propellants of rockets, chemical refining, steel and iron, petroleum, and paper industry. Oxygen enhances the combustion process in waste water treatment plants and in industries that manufacture glass, cement, nylon, polyvinyl chloride (PVC), antifreeze.

EVIDENCE AND IMPACT ON CLINICAL OUTCOMES

The survival benefit and improvement in pulmonary hemodynamics seen in Nocturnal Oxygen Therapy Trial (NOTT)[19] and the Medical Research Council (MRC) study, formed the foundation for Grade I recommendations for LTOT in chronic obstructive pulmonary disease (COPD) patients with severe hypoxemia [defined as PaO_2 ≤55 mm Hg or PaO_2 56–59 mm Hg plus either of the following: edema, P pulmonale on electrocardiography (ECG) and hematocrit ≥55%] by British and American thoracic societies recently concluded Long-term Oxygen Treatment Trial (LOTT trial) in stable COPD patients with moderate hypoxemia (defined as SpO_2 of 89–93%) at rest or exertion showed no benefit in mortality, COPD exacerbations, and COPD-related hospitalizations, quality of life, and lung functions making the use of LTOT in such subset of patients undesirable.

The duration of oxygen therapy (at least 15 hour/day) is the most important factor in the effectiveness of LTOT for survival benefit, on the contrary, the ANTADIR (Association Nationale de Traitement à Domicile des Insuffisants Respiratories-National Association for the Home Treatment of Chronic Respiratory Insufficiency at France) study for adherence to prescribed oxygen therapy conducted among 930 patients on LTOT, revealed only 45% of the patients actually received oxygen therapy for 15 hours or more per day. Poor compliance results in lower survival rates and increase unnecessary hospitalization. Patients on home oxygen therapy experience frequent and myriad problems associated with their oxygen equipment. A survey of 1,926 adult oxygen users found that 51% of respondents had problems due to equipment malfunction, delivery delays, insufficient support for travel with oxygen, physically unmanageable portable systems, and not enough tanks for oxygen outside the home.

Compared to portable oxygen concentrators (POCs), patients using LOX are likely to use oxygen for longer hours, go for more outings, and more likely to travel with oxygen. Ambulatory COPD patients are able to walk more effectively with portable LOX. The need for high flows drives the preference of LOX over a POC in patients with interstitial lung disease. A prospective, randomized multicenter trial comparing POC with LOX during a 6-month period showed significant differences in favor of the LOX in the following dimensions: physical function, ambulation, social interaction, and total sickness impact profile (SIP) score.

CONCLUSION

Liquid oxygen confers distinct storage, transport, and portability characteristics to home oxygen therapy. Cryogenic liquids have unique storage specifications mandating use of double-layered, thermal-insulated vacuum flasks (Dewar) and VIE vaporizers. LOX production occurs at a gigantic scale and in purest form by cryogenic fractional distillation of air in the Linde double column ASUs. Compared to POC and portable oxygen cylinders, LOX addresses the challenges of home oxygen therapy by meeting the oxygen needs at all activity levels, compact size, easy portability encouraging active lifestyle, pulmonary and physical rehabilitation. In contrast to traditional oxygen delivery equipment, patient friendly LOX equipment improves patient adherence to prescribed duration of oxygen therapy with potential to improve survival, quality of life, and exercise tolerance. LOX is best suitable for patients who have active lifestyle, continue to work outside their home, and require flow rates >5 L/min.

SUGGESTED READING

1. Air Products and Chemicals, Inc., 2015 (38983) https://www.airproducts.com/-/media/airproducts/files/en/900/900-13-078-us-liquid-oxygen-afetygram-6.pdf?la=en&hash=186006835357D54E196DF13FF41DB3B4
2. CAIRE. HELiOS Reservoirs for home oxygen therapy. User manual. [online] Available from http://files.caireinc.com/Manuals/21157307.pdf [Last accessed June, 2022].
3. Government of India. Guidance note on liquid medical oxygen (LMO) storage tanks. [online] Available from http://nhm.gov.in/New_Update-2021-22/PIP/ECRP-II/Guidance_Note_on_LMO_Storage_Tanks.pdf [Last accessed May, 2022].
4. Hardavella G, Karampinis I, Frille A, Sreter K, Rousalova I. Oxygen devices and delivery systems. Breathe (Sheff). 2019;15(3):e108-e116.
5. Jacobs SS, Lindell KO, Collins EG, Garvey CM, Hernandez C, McLaughlin S, et al. Patient perceptions of the adequacy of supplemental oxygen therapy. Results of the American Thoracic Society Nursing Assembly Oxygen Working Group Survey. Ann Am Thorac Soc. 2018;15(1):24-32.
6. Jacobs SS. Clinician strategies to improve the care of patients using supplemental oxygen. Chest. 2019;156(3):619-28.
7. McCoy RW. Options for home oxygen therapy equipment: storage and metering of oxygen in the home. Resp Care. 2013;58:65-85.
8. Soni NN, Maheshwari DG. Current regulation of medical gases in India and future aspects. Int J Drug Regul Aff. 2018;6(1):35-40.
9. World Health Organization. (2020). Oxygen sources and distribution for COVID-19 treatment centres. [online] Available from https://www.who.int/publications-detail/oxygen-sources-and-distribution-for-covid-19-treatment-centres [Last accessed June, 2022].

Oxygen Concentrators

CHAPTER 5

Khalid Ismail Khatib, Sameer V Kulkarni, Subhal B Dixit

INTRODUCTION

Oxygen concentrators are the main source of high fractional oxygen (FiO_2) supplementation to patients at home. They can also be used in hospitals or in ambulances. Oxygen concentrators are also used in some industries such as pharmaceutical companies, water treatment and glass manufacturing companies, and commercial airlines.

HISTORY

Oxygen concentrators were first invented in the 1950s but their real use started from the 1970s when the requirement of home oxygen (O_2) increased in patients of chronic obstructive pulmonary disease (COPD), obstructive sleep apnea (OSA), etc. Initially, oxygen concentrator machines were bulky and could give an output of only 1–5 L/min, which corresponds to 0.3–0.5% of FiO_2. But since the last 10–15 years, with the ongoing biomedical research and advancements in chemical substances, the adsorbents used in medical oxygen concentrators improved. Therefore, machines became smaller in size and could also give an output of >10 L/min of O_2 reaching a FiO_2 >0.9.

MECHANISM OF ACTION

A typical oxygen concentrator takes in atmospheric air (which contains 74% of nitrogen and 21% of O_2), removes a large amount of nitrogen from it, and supplies O_2-enriched gas (high FiO_2 of around 50%). Atmospheric nitrogen is removed with the help of nanosize zeolite adsorption technique. There are two techniques for the adsorption process, depending on the physical principle used: pressure swing adsorption (PSA) and temperature swing adsorption. Pressure swing adsorption process is preferred as it is heatless and faster.

Zeolites are preferred for PSA systems due to the following properties:
- Ability to discriminate between different gases
- Large specific surface area
- High porosity.

TYPES OF OXYGEN CONCENTRATOR

Oxygen concentrators may be stationary or portable **(Figs. 1 and 2) (Table 1)**.

Oxygen concentrators supply O_2 in the form of pulses (bolus of O_2 delivered at the beginning of inspiration) or a continuous supply of O_2.

COMPONENTS OF AN OXYGEN CONCENTRATOR (FIG. 3)

- Mechanism to compress air (air compressor)
- Area to store nitrogen-removing substance [multiple cylinders (two or more) filled with zeolite pellets or beads]
- Pressure-equalizing reservoir
- Area to store enriched air
- Valves/tubes.

CHAPTER 5: Oxygen Concentrators

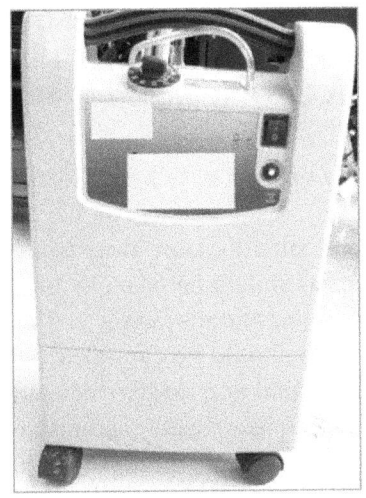

Fig. 1: Stationary oxygen concentrator.

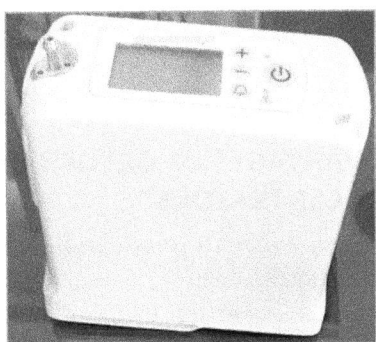

Fig. 2: Portable oxygen concentrator.

TABLE 1: Types of oxygen concentrators and their characteristics.		
Characteristics	*Stationary*	*Portable*
Weight	10 kg	4–5 kg
Electricity source	Run-on AC (Hence required to be plugged in the main electric socket)	Run-on AC or DC (Hence can run on the wall socket as well as other sources such as car electric socket)
Portability	Not easy to move	Extremely easy to move
Patient mobility	Better for sedentary patients	Better for patients who prefer an active lifestyle

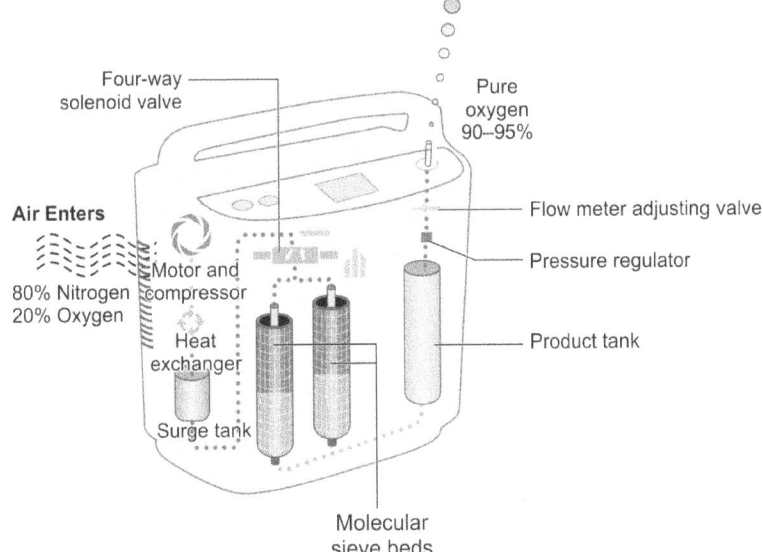

Fig. 3: Various components of an oxygen concentrator.

INDICATIONS

- Patients requiring long-term oxygen therapy (LTOT) for medical diseases such as COPD, OSA, and interstitial lung disease
- Patients requiring O_2 therapy for >1.4 h/day
- Patients on LTOT who prefer a more active lifestyle (portable oxygen concentrators).

ADVANTAGES OF OXYGEN CONCENTRATORS

- Oxygen concentrators can be used at home/hospital where the requirement of patient O_2 is less (less FiO_2).
- No need of frequent changes and replenishment like oxygen cylinders.
- Can be used in industries such as pharmaceutical companies, water treatment and glass manufacturing companies, and commercial airlines.
- More economical and cost-effective.
- Safe to use as there are less chances of leakage, cylinder blast or fire.
- Portable and can be used in military and disastrous situations.
- Had a great use in the COVID-19 pandemic all over the world, especially in patients who required O_2 at home.

DISADVANTAGES OF OXYGEN CONCENTRATORS

- Require electricity for their functioning. Hence, backup electricity generator may be needed during power outage.
- Require regular servicing.

SAFETY PRECAUTIONS FOR HOME USERS OF OXYGEN CONCENTRATORS

Oxygen concentrators are a fire hazard and must be kept away from fire, including cigarettes.

These must be kept away from water. Precautions should be taken by the patient during bathing and showering.

Patients should be careful while using aerosol products near oxygen concentrators as aerosol products are highly flammable.

CONCLUSION

Oxygen concentrators are a reliable and relatively economical device for LTOT. They are used to supply LTOT for patients requiring O_2 for more than 1.4 hours per day as they turn out to be more economical when compared to compressed oxygen cylinders.

SUGGESTED READING

1. Hardavella G, Karampinis I, Frille A, Sreter K, Rousalova I.. Oxygen devices and delivery systems. Breathe (Sheff). 2019;15(3):e108-16.
2. Jackson M, Shneerson J. An evaluation of the use of concentrators for domiciliary oxygen supply for less than 8 h day-1. Respir Med. 1998;92(2):250-5.
3. Pan M, Omar HM, Rohani S. Application of Nanosize Zeolite Molecular Sieves for Medical Oxygen Concentration. Nanomaterials (Basel). 2017;7(8):195.

Oxygen Hazards and Safety

CHAPTER 6

Deven Juneja, Prashant Nasa, Sahil Kataria

INTRODUCTION

Oxygen is necessary for survival and oxygen therapy is prescribed in most of the hospitalized patients as a part of their treatment regimen. However, like any other prescription drug, oxygen therapy may also be associated with side effects or toxicity. Even transportation, handling, storage, and delivery of oxygen may be associated with some harmful effects and hence oxygen is classified as a "hazardous material" by the occupational safety and health standards. All the personnel, including critical care physicians and anesthetists, who frequently handle and deliver oxygen, must be aware of the potential hazards of oxygen and the safety precautions required.

OXYGEN THERAPY IN HOSPITALS

Certain hospital areas are more vulnerable as compared to others. These areas are generally acute care areas such as emergency rooms, intensive care units, and operation theaters (OT), as all the three components to ignite the fire (the fire triangle), i.e., fuel, oxidizer, and heat, are in abundance **(Fig. 1)**. Even if one of these components is removed, the fire will stop propagating. Even though other components are also important, the use of electrocautery (heat), surgical drapes (fuel), and an open oxygen delivery system (oxidizer) have been most commonly implicated in OT fires.

Fig. 1: The fire triad.

Fuel:
- Alcohol-based solutions
- Gauzes
- Paper/files
- Wooden furniture/cabinets
- Clothing, sheets, drapes

Heat:
- Cautery
- Defibrillators
- Laser
- Drills
- High intensity lights

Oxidizer:
- Oxygen
- Nitric oxide
- Hyperbaric chamber

HAZARDS OF OXYGEN

Oxygen is noninflammable, but obviously, it is an oxidizer and is capable of causing or intensifying the fire. As oxygen is colorless, odorless, and tasteless, it is difficult to recognize that the environment is oxygen-enriched. In an oxygen-enriched environment, materials catch fire much easily because their inflammable range expands and the lowest temperature required to ignite without any spark or flame (autoignition temperature) starts to drop. Even materials, which are generally not easily combustible, such as metals, can ignite. In an oxygen-enriched environment, it is also impossible to extinguish a flame. Any source of heat, even that arising from friction generated by poorly functioning oxygen apparatus, can initiate a fire in such an environment. Easily combustible material burns faster and hotter in an oxygen-enriched environment, which may lead to a "kindling chain" reaction and a rapid spread of fire.

As the oxygen cylinders contain compressed gas under pressure, there is also a risk of explosion if they become heated. The common causes of fire and explosion related to oxygen include: creation of oxygen-enriched environment due to oxygen leak **(Box 1)**; using materials incompatible with oxygen; using equipment not designed to carry or deliver oxygen; and careless or incorrect use of oxygen apparatus.

SAFETY MEASURES

Several measures are essential to avoid any hazards associated with the supply, storage, transportation, and delivery of oxygen in the hospital environment **(Table 1)**. A safety checklist must be prepared and regular checks should be conducted at various points of oxygen use.

Hazard Analysis

It is prudent to conduct a fire hazard analysis in areas where oxygen is stored or used.

BOX 1: Causes of oxygen enrichment.
- Leaks from poorly maintained or damaged hoses, pipes, and valves
- Leaks from loose or poor connections/joints
- Deliberate or accidental opening of valves
- Improperly closed valves after use
- Using an excess of oxygen
- Poorly ventilated areas where oxygen is being used
- Misuse of oxygen, e.g., for air enrichment or dusting

TABLE 1: Safety measures to prevent oxygen hazards.

Oxygen cylinders	• Specialized cylinders constructed as per the recommendations • Legibly marked with the name of the gas • Markings should not be easily removable
Cylinder connections	• Should comply with the national/international recommendations • Should have a valve protection cap or cover
Storage of oxygen cylinders	• Stored in a well-ventilated, well-protected dry location • Protected from sunlight • Especially assigned area • Kept away from sources of heat • Kept away from combustible fuel/oil • Kept away from electric circuits
Transportation and handling of cylinders	• Do not use oily hands or gloves • Close the valves • Remove regulators and place valve caps
Oxygen delivery	• Specialized pipes and tubing to be used • Minimum joints or bents in the pipes • Open the valve slowly • Periodic cleaning of the pipes • Periodic check for any leaks
Personnel	• Authorized and trained personnel should handle the filling/refilling of cylinders • Periodic training and audit • Judicious use of oxygen

Such an analysis should be conducted at the initial stage and at frequent intervals. The analysis should identify the proper area where oxygen will be stored or used, materials used for the construction of oxygen apparatus, likelihood of ignition, and the safety measures to be instituted in case of fire **(Box 2)**.

Oxygen Storage

Oxygen should be stored and transported in especially designed containers or cylinders. Cylinders should be chained or held in such a way that they do not fall or hit each other. The connections should also be as per the recommended guidelines and have proper valve protection. These cylinders should be stored in the designated areas and clear off the walkways and staircases. These areas should be well-lighted, ventilated and protected, and away from any combustible agents or sources of heat. Direct heat from the sunlight should be avoided. The distance between oxygen cylinders and other fuel-gas cylinders or inflammable agents (oil or grease) should be at least 20 feet (6.1 meters) and/or separated by a noncombustible barrier that is at least 5 feet (1.5 meters) high with a fire-resistance rating of at least one-half hour. If oxygen is stored or used in poorly ventilated or confined areas, it is advisable to use oxygen monitoring equipment.

Oxygen Transportation

Oxygen cylinders should be transported in custom-built trolleys. During handling and transporting oxygen, avoid touching the cylinder with oily or greasy hands or gloves. In addition, the cylinders should be adequately separated from each other, ensuring that they do not strike violently with each other. During transportation, valve caps should be in place and regulators should be removed. Valves should be closed when the cylinders are not in use and during transport. Even when the cylinders are empty, these valves should be closed. If the valves are stuck, do not force them open using a hammer or a wrench and the supplier should be informed.

Oxygen Delivery

As per the manufacturer's instructions, proper connections and apparatus should be used. Cylinders should not be operated without an oxygen regulator. Even the gauges on oxygen regulators should be periodically checked and marked with "use no oil" **(Fig. 2)**. No one should tamper with the markings, connections, and safety devices of the cylinders.

The gas piping and fittings should be in accordance with the national guidelines and periodically checked and serviced. Stainless steel or copper alloys should be used if the piping carries oxygen at pressures above 700 psi (4.8 MPa). A pressure-measuring and -regulating device should be employed at each station outlet to detect any changes in pressure or the development of leaks.

> **BOX 2:** Components of fire hazard analysis.
> - Analysis of specific oxygen-enriched environment
> - Materials of construction for storage, transportation, and delivery of oxygen
> - *Likelihood of ignition:* Sources of heat, friction, and fire
> - Effects of fire

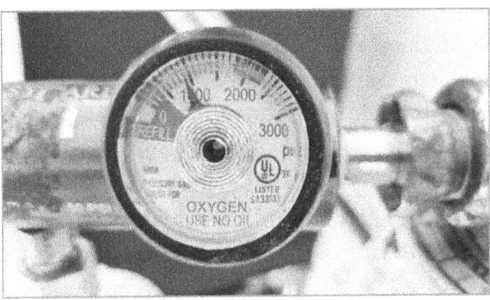

Fig. 2: Oxygen regulator.

Using closed oxygen delivery systems can reduce oxygen enrichment. Oxygen piping and tubing should have minimal bents and joints, to prevent any breaks or leaks. Oxygen piping and tubing must be regularly cleaned as even small contaminants or debris can catch fire when under pressure. Cleaning of oxygen pipes and tubes should be done using cleaning solutions which would not react with oxygen such as caustic soda or trisodium phosphate. Oxygen tubing or pipes should be kept in good condition and periodic leak tests must be performed using a specific spray or liquid solution.

While starting oxygen, valves should be opened slowly, as opening them rapidly can cause momentarily high oxygen velocity, generating frictional heat and precipitating fire.

Personnel

Authorized and trained personnel should handle the filling and refilling of cylinders and regular training and audit of all personnel involved in handling and delivery of oxygen should be conducted. Physicians should ensure judicious use of oxygen and should also be trained for fire control and evacuation in case of any fire.

Oxygen Leaks

In case of oxygen leaks, all personnel should be evacuated and the area should be sealed and secured. All sources of ignition should be eliminated and the area should be ventilated to ensure rapid gas dispersal. All combustible items should be removed from the vicinity. If possible, try to stop the flow of gas. If there is any leakage from the cylinder or valves, the valve should be closed immediately. However, if the leakage persists, the cylinder should be immediately taken outdoors and slowly emptied.

Fire alarms must be installed in all areas where oxygen is used or stored. Fire extinguishers should be placed in carefully selected sites and the hospital personnel should be trained regarding their location and to use them properly. Emergency alarm and evacuation plans for the patients and the healthcare workers should be in place, in case of a fire. Regular audits and fire drills should be conducted to ensure compliance and address any deficiencies.

■ DOMICILIARY OXYGEN THERAPY

Domiciliary oxygen is frequently prescribed to patients requiring long-term oxygen therapy. Hazards of oxygen must also be explained to the relatives or patients when domiciliary oxygen is prescribed. In addition, all safety precautions must be explained in detail and it should be emphasized that oxygen to be used and stored in well-ventilated areas. Family members should be asked to refrain from smoking or cooking in the nearby areas and it should be ensured that regular quality and safety checks are performed. At the time of initiation, a home oxygen risk assessment tool may be helpful in assessing the risk of domiciliary oxygen therapy.

■ CONCLUSION

Physicians handling oxygen must be aware of the potential hazards associated with oxygen and how to use it safely. Improper storage, transport, or oxygen delivery may cause burns or trauma secondary to fire or explosion. All measures should be instituted to ensure that the environment does not become oxygen-enriched by proper use of oxygen apparatus. In addition, areas where oxygen is stored or used should be adequately ventilated and there should be no heat or fire sources. Hazard risk analysis must be done at initiation and at regular intervals to ensure that oxygen is stored and used safely.

SUGGESTED READING

1. Apfelbaum JL, Caplan RA, Barker SJ, Connis RT, Cowles C, Ehrenwerth J, et al; American Society of Anesthesiologists Task Force on Operating Room Fires. Practice advisory for the prevention and management of operating room fires: an updated report by the American Society of Anesthesiologists Task Force on Operating Room Fires. Anesthesiology. 2013;118(2):271-90.
2. Cooper BG. Home oxygen and domestic fires. Breathe (Sheff). 2015;11(1):4-12.
3. Jones TS, Black IH, Robinson TN, Jones EL. Operating room fires. Anesthesiology. 2019;130(3):492-501.
4. Kelly FE, Bailey CR, Aldridge P, Brennan PA, Hardy RP, Henrys P, et al. Fire safety and emergency evacuation guidelines for intensive care units and operating theatres: for use in the event of fire, flood, power cut, oxygen supply failure, noxious gas, structural collapse or other critical incidents: Guidelines from the Association of Anaesthetists and the Intensive Care Society. Anaesthesia. 2021;76(10):1377-91.
5. Oxygen use in the workplace: fire and explosion hazards. [online] Available from https://www.hse.gov.uk/pubns/indg459.pdf. [Last accessed June, 2022].

Oxygen Audit

CHAPTER 7

Rahul Pandit

INTRODUCTION

Medical oxygen is a drug but unfortunately, its use is extensively associated with problems such as no prescription or proper protocol in hospitals, ambulances, and at home. There is no doubt that it is the most important gas, which is an absolute necessity in several medical conditions. The need for oxygen was never before felt so severely as it was during the second wave of COVID-19 in India in the summer of 2021. The demand which escalated due to a sudden increase in COVID-19 cases and COVID-19 acute respiratory distress syndrome (ARDS) patients, actually, was a wake-up alarm for a rude reality that we had taken availability of oxygen for granted and there was no real planning for a situation where there would be a scarcity of it. This led to a world and national outcry; the highest authorities took cognizance of it. This led to the concepts of oxygen stewardship and oxygen audit.

OXYGEN ECOSYSTEM

To complete an audit, we need to understand the oxygen ecosystem and oxygen stewardship. Oxygen ecosystem involves devices, instruments, and equipment used from producing oxygen to supplying it to the patient as well as for monitoring the oxygen levels. The oxygen ecosystem includes sources of oxygen production, its distribution, regulation, delivery, and patient-monitoring.

These are the multiple touch points where the possibility of an audit and improvement is seen.

OXYGEN STEWARDSHIP

The entire oxygen stewardship program is hospital-based and starts with demand projections of oxygen. We will study the following projection formulae for a 100-bed hospital, with 25 intensive care unit (ICU) beds with high oxygen demand.

Formulae to calculate the oxygen requirement:
- Per bed in L/min
- Allocation for 100-bed hospital with 25% ICU beds for ease of calculation

  Oxygen requirement calculated on L/min:
  - Each Bed- Ventilator/HFNC flow up to 60 L/min at an FiO_2 of 60% OR
  - On NIV will need maximum 30L/min flow at a similar FiO_2
  - Each oxygen bed will need an average of 10 L/min of oxygen.

Oxygen requirement for a 100-bed tertiary care hospital with 25% (25) ICU beds on full occupancy:
- Eight-bed ventilator at 80% FiO_2 = 8 × 30 = 240 L/min
- 10 NIV or HFNC at 70% FiO_2 = 10 × 30 = 300 L/min
- Four non-rebreather masks at 15 L/min = 4 × 15 = 60 L/min
- Three Hudson masks at 10 L/min = 3 × 10 = 30 L/min

- Wards and operating rooms 20 beds at 5 L/min = 20 × 5 = 100 L/min
- Total/min oxygen requirement = 240 + 300 + 60 + 30 + 100 = 730 L/min
- Daily requirement = 730 × 60 (min) × 24 (h) = 10,51,200 L/day ~ 10.5 lakh liters of gaseous oxygen per day
- 1 L of liquid oxygen produces 861 L of gaseous oxygen.
- Hence 10,51,200 L will be produced by 1051200/861 = 1,220 L of liquid oxygen per day.
- This equates to 1.39 MT of oxygen per day.
- With leaks at delivery circuits/mask/wastage/valves/pipes, around 5% extra will need to be added.
- The final requirement for a 100-bed hospital with 25 ICU beds on 100% capacity will be 1.39 + 0.06 = 1.45 MT per day.

This formula gives a baseline for the oxygen requirement for a 100-bed hospital with a very high demand. As per the situation, clinical cases, and case load, the requirement can be tweaked from this formula.

OXYGEN AUDIT AT THE HOSPITAL LEVEL

- *Oxygen Stewardship Program:*
  - Appoint oxygen stewarts who preach and practice rational use of oxygen across hospitals. (Educate all the staff about oxygen prescription and targets, develop "oxygen champion doctor/nurse" to monitor and audit ICU oxygen usage.)
  - Appoint oxygen audit committee—monitors oxygen use/supply and projected demand over the next 24 hours.
  - Give oxygen to patients who need it as a prescription, mentioning the flow rate and saturation targets.
- Turn off oxygen when patients do not need it.
- Minimum oxygen to be used to keep saturation within range.
- Use an appropriate mask/device to deliver oxygen.
- Change the target oxygen saturation to 92–94% in wards where there is intermittent monitoring.
- Use awake-prone ventilation to improve oxygen saturation. Use CARP (COVID awake repositioning and proning) protocol, which has shown to improve oxygenation.
- Taper oxygen quickly to minimum required to keep the saturation level to 92–94%.
- Use a nonrebreather mask with 8–10 L/min-flow for saving oxygen or use continuous positive airway pressure (CPAP) or bilevel positive airway pressure (BIPAP) machines that use less oxygen wherever possible.
- Careful/judicious use of high flow nasal oxygen (HFNO) machines as they use a very large quantity of oxygen, sometimes up to 80 L/min.
- Regulated use of HFNO—such as noncompliant patient to NIV/avoid intubation/patient difficult to prone on NIV (e.g., obese).
- Patients should be managed on NIV with minimum FiO_2 required to keep saturation between 92 and 94%.
- Use CARP protocol along with NIV to have effective use of oxygen.
- On invasive ventilator, aim for a saturation of 88–92% only or a PaO_2 of 55–65 mm Hg.
- Prone patients on invasive ventilation to improve oxygenation
- Cancel all routine surgeries and routine admissions to the hospital. This will save a significant amount of oxygen.
- Fix all leaking oxygen outlets, valves, and pressure gauge. Also, make sure that

oxygen-flow meters are off when the patient does not need oxygen.
- Form an oxygen audit committee in the hospital that would be responsible for all oxygen usage in the hospital.
- Oxygen concentrators: Rural areas and hospitals to use oxygen concentrators for patients who need up to 5 L/min of oxygen. This will save around 5–7% oxygen usage.

MONITORING OXYGEN NEED AT THE HOSPITAL LEVEL

- Oxygen monitoring committee should be set up in every hospital, consisting of an additional MS, head of ICU, anesthesia, respiratory medicine/internal medicine, and nursing superintendent.
- A monitoring team to be available round the clock (one duty nurse and one duty technician) to ensure proper assessment and possible steps to conserve oxygen such as closure of valve during no use and no leakage.
- To follow the guidelines for the target of oxygen saturation. The monitoring team should be vigilant and do target audits.
- Facility inspection every 2 months in detail to look at the pipes, valves etc., and carry necessary repairs.

MONITORING OXYGEN NEEDS AT THE STATE LEVEL

- Creation of an oxygen grid with 10–12 regional production and storage hubs with state and district storage spokes. Long haul connectivity through rail from the production hub to the storage hubs, with the last mile connectivity as a spoke model transported by trucks. The liquid medical oxygen (LMO) production hubs should be so located that the transport distance, even by rail, is <12–24 hours.
- Create a dashboard including health-facility-wise real-time data on the available infrastructure, beds, and actual oxygen consumption. The dashboard should be updated regularly.
- Tanker movement should be effectively managed and closely monitored from dispatch to recipient hospitals by respective states/UTs. For this, internet of things (IoT), GPS and other IT-based tools can be used to track each tanker.
- Ensure enough number of geographically distributed emergency reserve storage points to supply oxygen to hospitals, in case of SOS. Information on this should be widely disseminated, including contact numbers, names, and designations of the officers-in-charge.
- Each state should have access to reserve tankers to meet demand/supply mismatch.
- Allocation of tankers to the states during a pandemic may be taken over by the central government. Besides, to meet the urgent need of additional tankers, the government should continue to use the ISO containers.
- Once tankers are allocated to a state, they should manage the filling and distribution of oxygen to the urban and rural areas.

At the central government level, what should be the plan? The scenario would include routine distribution and audit and also an increase in demand and its projections.
- Effective communication to mitigate the request for more oxygen by the facilities than their actual requirement.
- The supply plan of oxygen to the high-burden states should be dynamic, based on the caseload and projection of cases. It should be reviewed in real time and changed as per requirement.
- A shifting demand: Some of the states need to shed their allocations as new allocations are made to other states.

- A supply chain expert may be involved [from supply chain organizations or Indian Institutes of Management (IIMs)] to give pragmatic inputs on oxygen supply throughout the country. There should be a system-based design for supply chain management.
- Creation of war room for real-time monitoring during any emergent situations, and it should be institutionalized. War room will monitor the movement of tankers, managing oxygen demand, its consumption and distribution in a real time, dynamic, and transparent manner. (During normal times there will not be the need for such a war room since the oxygen supply to the hospitals is done by manufacturers and suppliers as part of commercial arrangement.)
- A senior officer should be the head of the war room and its complete functioning, including distribution.
- Routine work should also be included in calculating the need and distribution of oxygen.
- As the rural hospitals are dependent on cylinders and concentrators (non-LMO sources), there may be a need to shift pressure swing adsorption (PSA) plants toward vulnerable areas. Cylinder turnaround time also needs to be efficient. An adequate number of cylinders must be kept as a buffer. The rural and semi urban areas' preparation should be prioritized henceforth.
- Concentrators should be used in COVID-care centers in rural areas and district hospitals where patients need 5 L/min oxygen, thereby saving about 5–7% oxygen usage.
- Oxygen cylinder filling and storage in rural areas are important. Hence, central filling stations should be considered in districts/rural areas.
- For smaller villages, liquid oxygen cylinders of 250 L may be considered to be parked for 10–12-bed facilities. Similar arrangements may be made for other villages as well.
- All oxygen cylinders to have radio frequency identification (RFID) tagging to make it easier to identify and track them.
- It is recommended that portable oxygen concentrators should be encouraged for home-care as a part of home-care packages and oxygen cylinders should be used in hospitals.
- We should have strategic reserves of oxygen for the country to cover 2–3 weeks' consumption, similar to the arrangement made for petroleum products. Similarly, all hospitals should have a buffer capacity for emergencies.
- There should be a strategy to manufacture oxygen locally or in the neighborhood for the big cities to fulfil at least 50% of their LMO demand, as road transportation is vulnerable. All metro cities to be made oxygen-independent, with at least 100 MT storage in the city itself.

CONCLUSION

The most important aspect to understand is that it is very easy to take our natural resources for granted. However, to conserve them and do a periodic check of their optimal production, distribution and use comprise a challenging task. The process is often dynamic and needs to be updated on a periodic basis.

SUGGESTED READING

1. Boyle M, Wong J. Prescribing oxygen therapy. An audit of oxygen prescribing practices on medical wards at North Shore Hospital, Auckland, New Zealand. N Z Med J. 2006;119(1238):U2080.
2. Kbar FA, Campbell IA Oxygen therapy in hospitalized patients: the impact of local guidelines. J Eval Clin Pract. 2006;12(1):31-6.

SECTION 2: Physiology and Monitoring of Oxygen Therapy

- **Physiology of Gas Exchange**
  Shilpushp Bhosale, Malini Joshi, Atul P Kulkarni

- **Goals of Oxygen Therapy**
  Vikram Damaraju, Inderpaul Sehgal

- **Drive to Breathe and Carbon Dioxide Retention**
  Prashant Nasa, Deven Juneja

- **Oxygen Transport**
  Ujwala Mhatre Ahluwalia, Kapil Borawake

- **Oxyhemoglobin Dissociation Curve**
  Srinivas Samavedam, Shabeer Ahmed Khan

- **Diffusion of Oxygen and its Applied Physiology**
  Srinivas Samavedam, Kiran Raghavendra Asrnanna

- **Pulse Oximetry: Undertsanding and Limitations**
  Kanwalpreet Sodhi, Manender Kumar

- **Venous and Arterial Blood Gas Analysis**
  Rajesh Pande, Maitree Pandey, Jitin Sharma

8. Physiology of Gas Exchange

CHAPTER

Shilpushp Bhosale, Malini Joshi, Atul P Kulkarni

INTRODUCTION

The primary function of the lungs is gas exchange, allowing oxygen (O_2) to be picked up from the atmosphere and carried to the cells and carbon dioxide (CO_2) to be released into the atmosphere. Diaphragm and intercostal muscle contraction drives the mechanics of ventilation. The lungs have around 300 million alveoli that take part in gas exchange. The air flowing into the alveoli have to overcome the airway resistance as well as elastic recoil of the lung and chest wall. The total alveolar surface area is around 140 m², allowing effective gas exchange. The alveolocapillary membrane, a 1 mm thin membrane, separates alveolar gas from blood pulmonary capillaries, across which gases diffuse by the process of simple diffusion, according to their partial pressure gradient. This process is influenced by the thickness of alveolar capillary membrane, diffusion coefficient of gas, surface area of membrane available for diffusion. The process, partial pressure of gases in alveoli and the blood and the affinity of hemoglobin for O_2 and CO_2. The affinity of hemoglobin itself varies depending on whether it is carrying O_2 or not. The pulmonary transit time is the time taken by the pulmonary capillary blood to flow around the alveoli (0.25–0.75 second).

Any unevenness in alveolar ventilation or pulmonary capillary blood flow alters gas exchange and this is described in terms of ventilation–perfusion (V/Q) mismatch or shunt. All lung diseases will cause significant V/Q mismatch depending on the physiological mechanisms and/or structural mechanisms in the disease. A shunt is the amount of deoxygenated blood returning from lungs without getting oxygenated. An increased shunt fraction (fraction of the total amount of blood passing through the lungs, i.e., proportion of cardiac output without getting oxygenated) can cause profound hypoxemia. Hypercapnia can occur if the shunt is massive. It is also important to note that in patients with increased shunt fraction, increasing the FiO_2 does not necessarily improve the PaO_2. As against this, oxygenation will improve if O_2 is supplemented in patients with V/Q mismatch. Since CO_2 is highly diffusible as compared to O_2 the alteration in V/Q ratios normally affect PaO_2 more than $PaCO_2$.

The dead space (VD/VT) is the fraction of the minute ventilation that does not take part in gas exchange. The anatomical dead space is the part of tidal volume (V_T) in the respiratory tree which carries air to the respiratory bronchioles and alveoli and does not take part in gas exchange. The physiological dead space is the air in the respiratory zone that does not take part in the gas exchange in addition to the anatomical dead space. VD/VT is normally around 30% of V_T and changes in V_T have a significant effect on dead space. For example, if the V_T is reduced to 400 mL from 500 mL, the VD/VT will increase to 38%, while with an increase in V_T to 2.0 L, the dead space will be reduced to 8%.

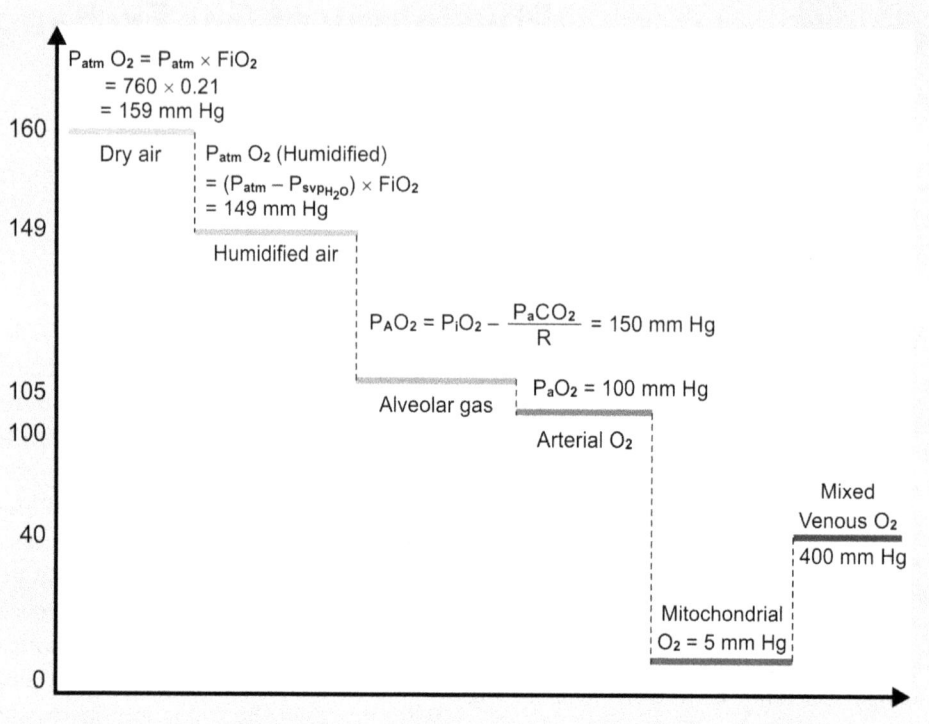

Fig. 1: Oxygen cascade.

The drop in partial pressure of O_2 from the atmospheric pressure (in the alveoli, PAO_2) through the blood (PaO_2) to the cellular level occurs in several steps and is called oxygen cascade **(Fig. 1)**. O_2 is transported in blood in two forms, bound to hemoglobin in the red blood cells (RBCs) and dissolved in plasma, whereas CO_2 is transported as dissolved in plasma, bound to hemoglobin, and in the form of HCO_3^-.

Diffusion of gases follow Henry's law, which states that for a constant temperature, the amount of dissolved gas in a liquid is directly proportional to the partial pressure of that gas (in contact with its surface). If it is a mixture of gases, then the amount of each gas dissolved will be directly proportional to its partial pressure. As the PAO_2 is higher than the PaO_2, there will be a net diffusion of O_2 into the blood. Diffusion equilibrium will be reached when the PaO_2 becomes equal to the PAO_2. Diffusion also depends on concentration gradient according to Fick's law of diffusion, i.e., rate of transfer of a substance (gas) across a membrane is directly proportional to the area of membrane, the diffusion constant (for that substance or gas), the partial pressure gradient across two compartments. And it is inversely proportional to the membrane thickness, surface area, and molecular weight of the substance (gas). The diffusion constant of a gas also depends on its solubility in blood (called blood–gas solubility). This is inversely proportional to the square root of the molecular weight. Dalton's law of gases suggests that the partial pressure of a mixture of gases is equal to the sum of the partial pressures exerted by each gas in the mixture.

TABLE 1: Etiology of hypoxemia and effect of supplemental oxygen.

Cause of hypoxemia	PAO$_2$	PAO$_2$-PaO$_2$ gradient as etiology of hypoxemia and effect of supplemental oxygen gradient	Response to supplemental O$_2$
Diffusion problem	Normal	Increased	May improve
Hypoventilation	Reduced	Normal	Improve
Decreased FiO2	Reduced	Normal	Improve
Low V/Q	Reduced	Normal	Improve
Shunt	Normal	Increased	Does not improve

(V/Q: ventilation–perfusion)

According to the fundamental principle of conservation of mass, the amount of O_2 diffusing in the pulmonary blood can be quantified as product of pulmonary blood flow and pulmonary venoarterial O_2 difference.

ALVEOLAR GAS EQUATION

Alveolar gas equation helps us to estimate partial pressure of O_2 in the alveoli (PAO$_2$). PAO$_2$ depends on the atmospheric PO$_2$, the alveolar ventilation, and the O_2 consumption.

$$PAO_2 = (P_{atm} - PH_2O) FiO_2 - PaCO_2/RQ,$$

where P_{atm} is atmospheric pressure (760 mm Hg, at sea level), PH$_2$O is saturated water vapor pressure (47 mm Hg at 37°C), PACO$_2$ is alveolar CO_2 tension (40 mm Hg assumed to be equal to arterial PCO$_2$), and RQ is the respiratory quotient (i.e., 0.8–1.0). Thus, a patient breathing air and 100% O_2 will have PAO$_2$ of 104 and 663 mm Hg, respectively.

$$PAO_2 = [(760 - 47) \times 1] - (40/0.8)$$

Thus, in normal patient receiving 100% FiO$_2$, increased O_2 reserve and therefore prolonged apnea time (without desaturation) during intubation will be present. However, it must be noted that in pathological conditions such as pneumonia, heart failure, etc., where diffusion is impaired, preoxygenation may not improve oxygenation. Any condition that can cause reduction in the alveolar O_2 (alveolar hypoventilation or high altitude) can lead to hypoxia. If hypoxia stimulates the respiratory center, the increase in respiratory rate will reduce PaCO$_2$, but if ventilatory response is blunted for some reason, hypercapnea will occur.

ALVEOLAR–ARTERIAL GRADIENT

The alveolar-arterial gradient for O_2 [the D(A-a) O_2 or PAO$_2$-PaO$_2$] is used to assess the diffusion across the alveolocapillary membrane and helps in diagnosing the cause of hypoxemia (Table 1). The normal PAO$_2$-PaO$_2$ gradient is 5-10 mm Hg, but progressively increases up to 25 mm Hg with increasing age. Unlike PAO$_2$, the PaO$_2$ is not calculated but measured. In normal conditions, PaO$_2$ is approximately given as [102 - (Age/3)] mm Hg, and the diffusion capacity for O_2 is approximately 21 mL/min/mm Hg at rest. Finally, the PAO$_2$ and PACO$_2$ are well maintained by complex neural regulation of alveolar ventilation. As the blood passes the alveolocapillary membrane, it gets rapidly oxygenated.

Bulk of O_2 is carried bound to hemoglobin and a very small portion (0.003 mL/dL/mm Hg or 3 mL/L) is in the dissolved form. The dissolved portion maintains the arterial O_2 tension (PaO$_2$ 100 mm Hg). Hemoglobin is a tetramer with four subunits, two α and two β, which form two identical αβ dimers, with heme group each. Heme groups are iron-containing molecules of protoporphyrin-IX with hydrophilic cores and hydrophobic external chains. The iron portion of heme molecule can switch between ferric (Fe^{3+}) and ferrous (Fe^{2+}) states, allowing it to participate in oxidation and reduction reactions. Hemoglobin takes only 0.25 second to become fully saturated, which is more than sufficient as the pulmonary transit time is 0.25–0.75 second.

OXYGEN CONTENT OF BLOOD

The O_2 content of the arterial (CaO_2) or venous (CvO_2) blood can be calculated using the formula

$$CaO_2 = [1.34 \times Hb\,(g\%) \times \%\,Saturation] + [0.0031 \times PaO_2]\,mL/dL$$

where PaO_2 is the partial pressure of O_2, Hb is the hemoglobin concentration, and % saturation is the O_2 saturation of the hemoglobin. Therefore, arterial O_2 content in 100 mL blood in a person with Hb of 15 g% (1 g Hb binds 1.34 when fully saturated), PaO_2 of 100, and 97.5% saturated would be 20 mL O_2/dL while in mixed venous blood with a PO_2 of 40 mm Hg and Hb saturation of 75% would be approximately 15 mL/dL.

OXYGEN DELIVERY AND CONSUMPTION

The O_2 delivery (DO_2) is the amount of O_2 delivered to the tissues per minute and is determined by the CaO_2 and the cardiac output per minute. The normal DO_2 in adults at rest is approximately 1,000 mL/min, (also known as oxygen flux, defined as amount of O_2 leaving the left ventricle/min). The O_2 consumption (VO_2) is the amount of O_2 consumed by tissues/minute and is the difference in the arterial and venous O_2 content. It is roughly around 250 mL/min at rest, i.e., $VO_2 = Q \times (CaO_2 - CvO_2)$. The oxygen extraction ratio (O_2ER) is the ratio of O_2 consumption to DO_2 and is 0.25 at rest, i.e., 25% of the O_2 delivered is taken up by the tissues:

$$O_2ER = VO_2/DO_2.$$

CONCLUSION

Understanding the physiology of gas exchange is critical to assess the severity and nature of gas exchange abnormalities and formulate strategies to treat patients with pulmonary and other critical pathologies.

SUGGESTED READING

1. Cardús J, Burgos F, Diaz O, Roca J, Barberà JA, Marrades RM, et al. Increase in pulmonary ventilation/perfusion inequality with age in healthy individuals. Am J Respir Crit Care Med. 1997;156(2 Pt 1):648-53.
2. Glenny RW. Determinants of regional ventilation and blood flow in the lung. Intensive Care Med. 2009;35:1833-42.
3. Janssens JP, Pache JC, Nic$_o$d LP. Physiological changes in respiratory function associated with ageing. Eur Respir J. 1999;13:197-205.
4. Lumb AB. Nunn's Applied Respiratory Physiology, 5th edition. Oxford: Butterworth-Heinemann; 2000.
5. Wagner PD, Laravuso RB, Uhl RR, West JB. Continuous distributions of ventilation-perfusion ratios in normal subjects breathing air and 100 per cent O_2. J Clin Invest. 1974;54(1):54-68.
6. West JB. State of the art: ventilation-perfusion relationships. Am Rev Respir Dis. 1977;116:919-43.

Goals of Oxygen Therapy

CHAPTER 9

Vikram Damaraju, Inderpaul Sehgal

INTRODUCTION

The cardinal goal of oxygen therapy is to improve tissue hypoxia. Tissue hypoxia is of the following types: (1) Anemic hypoxia (low hemoglobin, carbon monoxide poisoning); (2) Stagnant hypoxia (inadequate blood flow); (3) Histotoxic hypoxia (cyanide poisoning); and (4) Hypoxemic hypoxia [low PaO_2 in blood secondary to high altitude, alveolar hypoventilation, right-to-left shunts, diffusion impairment, and ventilation–perfusion (V/Q) mismatch]. However, oxygen delivery to the tissue depends not only on SaO_2 and PaO_2 but also on cardiac output and hemoglobin. Accordingly, it is pertinent to understand that oxygen therapy cannot correct all causes of tissue hypoxia (like shunts).

MEASURES OF TISSUE OXYGENATION

The differences in the regional blood flow to different organs lead to the nonuniform distribution of oxygen at the cellular level. The normal ranges of oxygen delivery index and oxygen uptake index are 520–570 $mL/min/m^2$ and 110–160 $mL/min/m^2$, respectively. The fraction of oxygen delivered at the capillary level taken up by tissues is the oxygen extraction ratio, usually about 20–30%. In critically ill patients, the oxygen delivery to the tissues varies widely between 150 and 1,000 $mL/min/m^2$, with an average value of 300 $mL/min/m^2$ (critical oxygen delivery). Ideally, PO_2 at the tissue level needs to be assessed for adequate oxygenation. However, the normal values are different for different tissues and are cumbersome to monitor routinely at the bedside.

Thus, clinical assessment (delayed signs of tissue hypoxia at the organ level: altered sensorium, decreased urine output, increased capillary refill time, and hemodynamic instability) and other measures of oxygen delivery and uptake are such as SaO_2, SpO_2, PaO_2, mixed venous O_2 saturation (SvO_2, requires central venous catheter), SaO_2–SvO_2 (dual oximetry: a measure of oxygen extraction), and the ratio of oxygen delivery to oxygen consumption are monitored for routine care. Some other measures of regional tissue oxygenation are gastric intramucosal pH, sublingual capnography, and near-infrared spectroscopy (NIRS) measures oxyhemoglobin, deoxyhemoglobin, cytochrome oxidase, and nuclear magnetic resonance spectrometry [adenosine triphosphate (ATP) and metabolites of oxidative phosphorylation]. Even though NIRS has evolved as potential tissue oximetry, threshold values have not been defined, and lack prediction studies with clinical outcomes.

SaO_2, PaO_2, and SpO_2

Hypoxemia is defined as a PaO_2 <60 mm Hg and a SaO_2 <90% in the arterial blood. The oxygen–hemoglobin dissociation curve depicts the relationship between SaO_2 of hemoglobin and PaO_2 of blood. The characteristic aspect of the curve is that PaO_2 drops rapidly when SaO_2 falls below 90%, reducing the oxygen delivery to the tissues. Another point to note is that, above a PaO_2 of 90 mm Hg (up to 700 mm Hg), the rise in SaO_2 flattens out (with a minimal increase in SaO_2 from 97 to 99%). Blood gas analysis of SaO_2 and PaO_2 is invasive, difficult, painful, and needs frequent arterial punctures. Pulse oximetric measurement of SpO_2 values lies within ±2% of SaO_2, is immediate, noninvasive, allows continuous monitoring, and is relatively inexpensive, making it a reliable alternative (potential limitations of pulse oximetry need to be considered) to SaO_2 and PaO_2 for monitoring oxygen therapy.

GOALS OF OXYGEN THERAPY

The main goal of oxygen therapy is to treat hypoxemia and prevent hyperoxemia. Hyperoxemia can lead to increased free radical generation and associated tissue damage, resorptive atelectasis, risk of hypercapnic respiratory failure in chronic obstructive pulmonary disease (COPD) patients, coronary vasoconstriction, and mortality. Furthermore, hyperoxemia can delay early recognition of deterioration by false reassurance. Closed-loop oxygen titration systems help maintain the SpO_2 targets set for a particular patient and prevent hyperoxemia.

LIBERAL OXYGEN THERAPY VERSUS CONSERVATIVE OXYGEN THERAPY

The terms liberal and conservative are relative, and the targets are not discrete. Higher oxygen targets increase the risk of exposure to hyperoxemia and overlooking potential desaturation events while having a theoretical benefit in subjects with severe anemia and hypotension. Lower oxygen targets may lead to intermittent or transient episodes of hypoxemia and risk of mesenteric ischemia.

The practice of oxygen therapy has been more liberal (till recently), which can result in hyperoxemia and its associated adverse outcomes. The Oxygen-ICU trial randomized 434 critically ill patients to either a conservative group (target: SpO_2 between 94 and 98%, PaO_2 between 70 and 100 mm Hg) or a conventional control group (target: SpO_2 between 97 and 100%, PaO_2 up to 150 mm Hg) and found lower mortality and reduced rates of shock, bacteremia and liver failure in the conservative arm. A meta-analysis by Chu et al. of oxygen therapy in acutely ill patients (some of the studies included patients who were not even hypoxemic, and saturation targets were not uniform between studies and heterogeneous population), found high mortality in subjects receiving liberal oxygen therapy (treatment arm with higher oxygen target) than those receiving conservative oxygen therapy (treatment arm with lower oxygen target). However, in the Liberal or Conservative Oxygen ($LOCO_2$) trial, where ARDS respiratory distress syndrome (ARDS) patients were randomized to a conservative arm (target: SpO_2 88–92%, PaO_2 55–70 mm Hg) or liberal arm (target: SpO_2 ≥96%, PaO_2 90–105 mm Hg), a worrsiome but not a significant increase in mortality and rates of mesenteric ischemia were noted in the conservative therapy arm, resulting in premature stoppage of trial. In the ICU-ROX study that included 1,000 mechanically ventilated subjects, the number of ventilator-free days and mortality were not different between the two arms [conservative arm (target SpO_2: 90–97%) and usual arm (target SpO_2: ≥91%, no predefined upper limit)]. However, in the subgroup analysis, patients with hypoxic ischemic encephalopathy treated with conservative oxygen had significantly higher ventilator-free days. The HOT-ICU (Handling Oxygenation Targets in the ICU) trial randomized 2,928 acute hypoxemic respiratory failure patients to target a PaO_2 of 60 mm Hg (lower oxygenation group) or 90 mm Hg (higher oxygenation group). There was no difference in mortality or new-onset shock, myocardial ischemia, stroke, or intestinal ischemic events in the two groups. A subsequent meta-analysis, including these recent trials, found no significant mortality difference between the two strategies.

There are several limitations to these randomized studies. Most of the trials had a heterogeneous population (stroke, sepsis, myocardial ischemia, traumatic brain injury, cardiac arrest, limb ischemia, and acute appendicitis). The inclusion of such patients can be argued by the fact that hyperoxemia has the physiological benefit of increasing PaO_2 and, therefore, tissue oxygenation in subjects with severe anemia and hypotension. However, these factors have not been accounted for in those trials, and supplementing oxygen to normoxic patients (median baseline SpO_2 was 94% in most of the trials) is not rational. Targeting supraphysiologic PaO_2 up to 150 mm Hg and SpO_2 between 97 and 100% in the liberal arm of the Oxygen-ICU trial could have resulted in higher mortality. The HOT-ICU and $LOCO_2$ trials are the only major studies including patients with hypoxemic respiratory failure. However, data from these studies are contrasting. Future studies may be required to include hypoxemic patients (only) not at risk of hypercapnia, with three arms (SpO_2 targets of 88–92%, 93–95%, 96–100%).

Based on the current evidence, we suggest using a target SPO_2 of 90–95% or a PaO_2 of ≥60 mm Hg should be maintained in those with acute hypoxemic respiratory failure.

Oxygen targets in those not at risk of hypercapnic respiratory failure: Considering the risk of hyperoxemia with liberal oxygen therapy, variable PaO_2 levels above a SpO_2 of 96%, the upper limit of the SpO_2 target is recommended to be ≤96%. Owing to the difference of ± 2% between SaO_2 and SpO_2 and a rapid fall in PaO_2 levels when SaO_2 falls below 90%, the lower limit of the SpO_2 target is recommended to be 92%.

Oxygen targets in those at risk of hypercapnic respiratory failure: Subjects with COPD, obesity, cystic fibrosis, neuromuscular disease, and thoracic deformities are at risk of hypercapnic respiratory failure with hyperoxemia. Subjects with COPD exacerbation and SpO_2 >92% at admission had increased mortality in an observational study. In a Cochrane review of oxygen therapy for acute exacerbation of COPD in the prehospital setting, the conservative oxygen therapy group had reduced mortality than the high flow treatment arm. Hence, SpO_2 targets for these subjects were recommended to be between 88 and 92%.

Oxygen targets in other conditions: The targets are similar for patients with acute coronary syndrome, stroke, and other neurological disorders, procedures involving conscious sedation, pregnancy, and during delivery of a child. The targets remain similar, though the data is sparse in paraquat poisoning and bleomycin-toxicity (increased risk of pulmonary fibrosis due to formation of reactive oxygen radicals). FiO_2 should remain high (100% or 15 L/min flow) during cardiopulmonary resuscitation (CPR) or when the pulse oximeter signal is not reliable in a patient with shock. However, after resuscitation and return of spontaneous circulation, SpO_2 targets should be between 92 and 96%. For subjects with carbon monoxide poisoning, FiO_2 should be 100% until the patient improves, independent of SpO_2.

To conclude, tissue hypoxia cannot be corrected by oxygen supplementation alone. There are several measures of oxygen delivery and utilization; however, none of them are ideal. The terms liberal and conservative treatments are not discrete, and the oxygenation targets are different in different subjects. The data from the previous studies is inconsistent, and future studies are required whether to target normal or supranormal PaO_2.

SUGGESTED READING

1. Barbateskovic M, Schjørring OL, Russo Krauss S, Jakobsen JC, Meyhoff CS, Dahl RM, et al. Higher versus lower fraction of inspired oxygen or targets of arterial oxygenation for adults admitted to the intensive care unit. Cochrane Database Syst Rev. 2019;2019(11):CD012631.
2. Barrot L, Asfar P, Mauny F, Winiszewski H, Montini F, Badie J, et al. Liberal or conservative oxygen therapy for acute respiratory distress syndrome. N Engl J Med. 2020;382(11): 999-1008.
3. Bickler P, Feiner J, Rollins M, Meng L. Tissue oximetry and clinical outcomes. Anesth Analg. 2017;124(1):72-82.
4. Chu DK, Kim LH, Young PJ, Zamiri N, Almenawer SA, Jaeschke R, et al. Mortality and morbidity in acutely ill adults treated with liberal versus conservative oxygen therapy (IOTA): a systematic review and meta-analysis. Lancet. 2018;391(10131): 1693-705.
5. Cumpstey AF, Oldman AH, Smith AF, Martin D, Grocott MP. Oxygen targets in the intensive care unit during mechanical ventilation for acute respiratory distress syndrome: a rapid review. Cochrane Database Syst Rev. 2020;9(9):CD013708.
6. Gottlieb J, Capetian P, Hamsen U, Janssens U, Karagiannidis C, Kluge S, et al. German S3 guideline: oxygen therapy in the acute care of adult patients. Respiration. 2022;101(2): 214-52.
7. Li L, Zhang Y, Wang P, Chong W, Hai Y, Xu P, et al. Conservative versus liberal oxygen therapy for acutely ill medical patients: a systematic review and meta-analysis. Int J Nurs Stud. 2021;118:103924.
8. O'Driscoll BR, Howard LS, Earis J, Mak V. British Thoracic Society guideline for oxygen use in adults in healthcare and emergency settings. BMJ Open Respir Res. 2017;4(1): e000170.

Drive to Breathe and Carbon Dioxide Retention

CHAPTER *Prashant Nasa, Deven Juneja*

INTRODUCTION

Lung is the primary organ that facilitates gas exchange between the circulatory system and the inspired air. Carbon dioxide (CO_2), a byproduct of the body's metabolism, plays a vital role in the body's homeostasis as a driver of respiration, blood buffer to regulate pH, and facilitates hemoglobin-bound oxygen delivery to the tissues. The blood levels of CO_2 are tightly regulated, and CO_2 elevation is caused by hypoventilation or a failure to remove excess CO_2. In this chapter, we will discuss the physiology of the respiratory drive and its role in CO_2 retention.

PHYSIOLOGY OF THE RESPIRATORY DRIVE AND CARBON DIOXIDE TRANSORT

The respiratory center of the brain is composed of three groups of neurons that are in the pons and the medulla oblongata of the brainstem **(Fig. 1)**. The medulla includes inspiratory

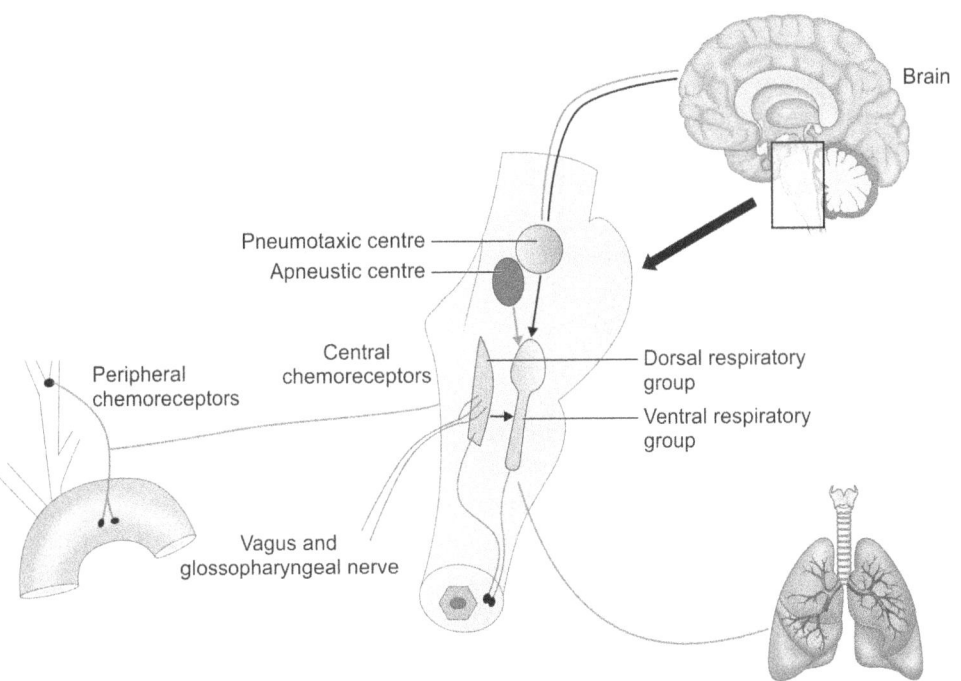

Fig.1: Respiratory centre.

dorsal and expiratory ventral respiratory group, and the pontine group which is subclassified into pneumotaxic and apneustic centers. The intercommunication between these neurons and inputs from the cerebral cortex, hypothalamus, chemoreceptors, and baroreceptors regulates the rate, depth, and rhythm of the respiration. The chemoreceptor reflex primarily supports the respiratory drive. There are two types of chemoreceptors: (1) Peripheral and (2) Central.

Peripheral chemoreceptors are located around the bifurcation of the common carotid arteries (carotid bodies) and along the aortic arch (aortic bodies). The chemoreceptors in the carotid bodies interact with the respiratory center via the glossopharyngeal cranial nerve and the aortic bodies through the vagus nerve. Peripheral chemoreceptors are triggered by hypoxemia (main stimulus), hypercapnia, and acidosis. A fall of 12% or more of inspired oxygen concentration [equivalent to partial pressure of oxygen (PaO_2) of 50–60 mm Hg] is required to drive ventilation.

Central chemoreceptors are located on the surface of the medulla and are separated from the blood through a semipermeable blood-brain barrier. The blood-brain barrier is permeable to molecular CO_2, which then dissociates into hydrogen (H^+) and bicarbonate (HCO_3^-) ions inside the cerebrospinal fluid (CSF). Central chemoreceptors are sensitive to a hypercapnic drop in the pH of the CSF compared to metabolic acidosis because of the impermeability of the blood-brain barrier to H^+ ions. Thus, central receptors are sensitive to changes in CO_2 or pH, while peripheral chemoreceptors are mainly sensitive to hypoxemia and play only a minor role in the respiratory drive.

CO_2 is transported in various forms inside the blood to the lung for removal. Most of the CO_2 (80–90%) is carried in the dissolved form as HCO_3^-. Carbon dioxide is 20 times more soluble in the plasma than oxygen. Around 5–10% of CO_2 is dissolved in plasma and around 5–10% is transported as bound to blood proteins or carbamino compounds (as carbaminohemoglobin). The affinity of hemoglobin for CO_2 and CO_2-carrying capacity in the blood is increased in the deoxyhemoglobin state, i.e., the Haldane effect **(Fig. 2)**. In tissues with low SpO_2, the CO_2 dissociation curve shifts to the left, permitting the loading of CO_2 to hemoglobin. The reverse happens in the lungs where offloading of CO_2 occurs in an oxyhemoglobin state—the reverse Haldane effect.

CARBON DIOXIDE RETENTION AND CLINICAL SIGNIFICANCE

Carbon dioxide retention or hypercapnia is defined as the partial pressure of CO_2 in the arterial blood ($PaCO_2$) >42 mm Hg. An arterial blood gas is required to evaluate patients with suspected hypercapnia.

The HCO_3^--CO_2 buffer system plays a vital role in regulating the blood-pH. The dissolved CO_2 in the blood is neutralized into weak carbonic acid (H_2CO_3). $H_2CO_3^-$ dissolution into H^+ and HCO_3^- is facilitated by carbonic anhydrase present in the erythrocytes.

$$CO_2 + H_2O \xrightarrow{\text{Carbonic anhydrase}} H_2CO_3 \rightarrow H^+ + HCO_3^-$$

In case of CO_2 retention, there is a rightward shift of the above equation, increasing the H^+ in the bloodstream, lowering the pH, and creating acidemia. In contrast, there is a leftward shift in the equation during hypocapnia, resulting in alkalemia.

The symptom of hypercapnia depends on the rate of increase in CO_2. The symptoms may be mild with chronic CO_2 retention, and in case

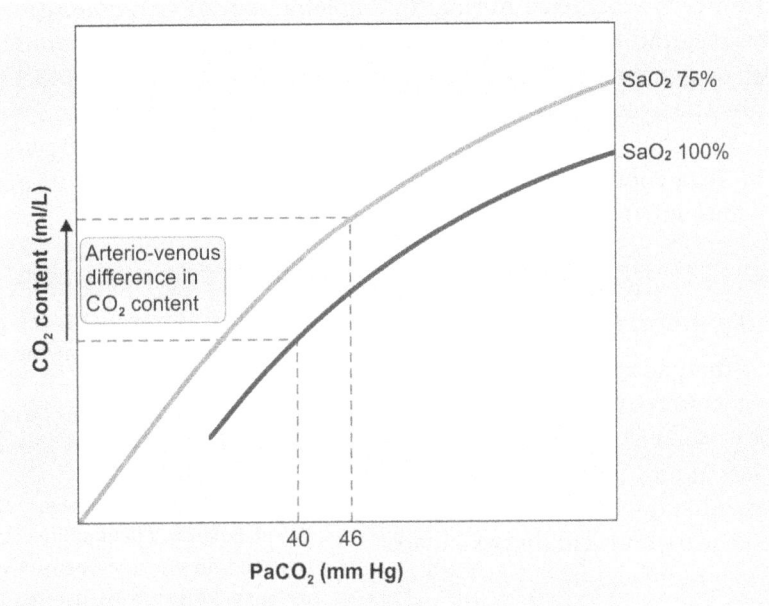

Fig. 2: Carbon dioxide-dissociation Curve.

of acute worsening, symptoms may rapidly progress to respiratory failure. The clinical presentation includes breathlessness, flushed skin, diaphoresis, tachycardia, confusion, headaches, dizziness, or a reduced level of consciousness. Both $PaCO_2$ and pH are essential for the severity of clinical presentation; for example, a pH of <7.3 in patients with acute exacerbation of chronic obstructive pulmonary disease (COPD) is more likely to require intensive care admissions.

Respiratory Drive and Carbon Dioxide Retention

Carbon dioxide retention is common in patients with exacerbations of COPD. However, uncontrolled oxygen administration to patients with COPD can cause a further and progressive increase in $PaCO_2$. Randomized controlled trials (RCTs) investigating different oxygen concentrations on the degree of CO_2 retention and clinical outcomes are lacking. However, the available evidence supports that a higher concentration is more likely to increase $PaCO_2$ than a low concentration. Titrating oxygen therapy to target peripheral oxygen saturation (SpO_2) of 88–92% can reduce the risk of hospital mortality when compared to high concentration oxygen therapy. An RCT found 2.4-fold increased risk of mortality with the use of prehospital high concentration oxygen in acute exacerbation of COPD compared to titrate oxygen therapy. The number needed to treat to prevent one death from high concentration oxygen was 14. Uncontrolled oxygen therapy can also lead to CO_2 retention in other disorders such as severe asthma, community-acquired pneumonia, obesity-hypoventilation syndrome, and acute respiratory distress syndrome.

Traditionally, it was believed that the elimination of hypoxic drive with uncontrolled oxygen administration causes CO_2 retention in patients with acute exacerbation of COPD. However, this was without any scientific evidence. Recent studies showed that patients with COPD exacerbation have normal to supranormal respiratory drive, and high-concentration oxygen therapy does not affect respiratory drive and ventilatory response to hypercarbia. The actual mechanism of CO_2 retention with high-concentration oxygen is ventilation/perfusion (V/Q) mismatch and the Haldane effect.

Ventilation/Perfusion Mismatch

The lungs of the patients with COPD are indeed dependent on hypoxic vasoconstriction in order to optimize gas exchange from progressive loss of lung volume. The uncontrolled oxygen therapy leads to the loss of hypoxic vasoconstriction and diverts blood flow to the poorly ventilated alveoli, increasing physiological dead space. This increases the V/Q mismatch and leads to CO_2 retention.

Haldane Effect

As mentioned above, oxyhemoglobin reduces the affinity toward CO_2, shifts the CO_2-dissociation curve toward the right, and increases $PaCO_2$. The Haldane effect contributes nearly one-fourth of CO_2 retention with high-concentration oxygen administration.

CONCLUSION

Respiratory drive is dependent on the chemoreceptors' reflex. Hypercapnia is the primary stimulus for central chemoreceptors and hypoxemia for peripheral chemoreceptors. CO_2 retention is caused by either hypoventilation or a failure to remove excess CO_2. The primary mechanism of CO_2 retention with high-concentration oxygen therapy in patients with acute exacerbation of COPD is the V/Q mismatch or the Haldane effect. Titrated oxygen therapy with an SpO_2 target of 88-92% can improve outcomes in patients with exacerbation of COPD.

SUGGESTED READING

1. Abdo WF, Heunks LM. Oxygen-induced hypercapnia in COPD: myths and facts. Crit Care. 2012;16(5):323.
2. Abdo WF, Heunks LM. Oxygen-induced hypercapnia in COPD: myths and facts. Crit Care. 2012;16(5):323.
3. Austin MA, Wills KE, Blizzard L, Walters EH, Wood-Baker R. Effect of high flow oxygen on mortality in chronic obstructive pulmonary disease patients in prehospital setting: randomised controlled trial. BMJ. 2010;341: c5462.
4. Brill SE, Wedzicha JA. Oxygen therapy in acute exacerbations of chronic obstructive pulmonary disease. Int J Chron Obstruct Pulmon Dis. 2014;9:1241-52.
5. Inkrott JC. Understanding hypoxic drive and the release of hypoxic vasoconstriction. Air Med J. 2016;35(4):210-1.
6. Patel S, Miao JH, Yetiskul E, Anokhin A, Majmundar SH. Physiology, Carbon Dioxide Retention. In: StatPearls [online]. Treasure Island (FL): StatPearls Publishing; 2022. Available from: https://www.ncbi.nlm.nih.gov/books/NBK482456/ [Last accessed June, 2022].
7. Rialp G, Raurich JM, Llompart-Pou JA, Ayestarán I. Role of respiratory drive in hyperoxia-induced hypercapnia in ready-to-wean subjects with COPD. Respir Care. 2015;60(3):328-34.

CHAPTER 11

Oxygen Transport

Ujwala Mhatre Ahluwalia, Kapil Borawake

INTRODUCTION

Oxygen is vital for survival and hemoglobin (Hb) is essential for oxygen transport to the tissues. In this chapter, we shall discuss diffusive and convective properties, artificial oxygen, and clinical applications.
1. Transfer of oxygen from atmosphere to lungs
2. Diffusion across alveoli to blood
3. Diffusion from blood to tissue
4. Utilization of oxygen in tissues, i.e., mitochondria

CONVECTIVE OXYGEN TRANSPORT

Convective oxygen transport includes oxygen uptake, content, delivery, and oxygen dissociation curve.

Oxygen Uptake in Blood

Oxygen diffuses through the alveolar capillary membrane by a partial pressure gradient and binds to Hb, forming oxyhemoglobin, and also gets dissolved in plasma. Hb, an allosteric protein, consists of four protein (globin) chains, to each of which is attached a heme moiety, an iron-porphyrin compound. Two pairs of globin chains exist within each Hb molecule **(Figs. 1A and B)**.

Hemoglobin A consists of two α- and two β-chains ($\alpha_2\beta_2$) and accounts for >95% of normal adult Hb. Other Hb types are hemoglobin A2, hemoglobin F (fetal), and hemoglobin S (seen in sickle cell disease). Up to four molecules of oxygen can bind to one Hb molecule and the shape of the globin chain is altered, leading to an overall change in the quaternary structure

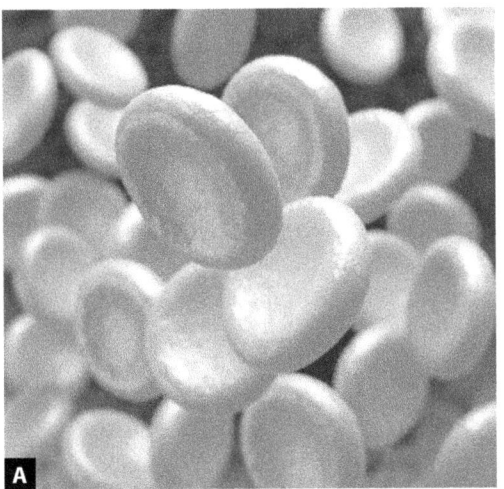
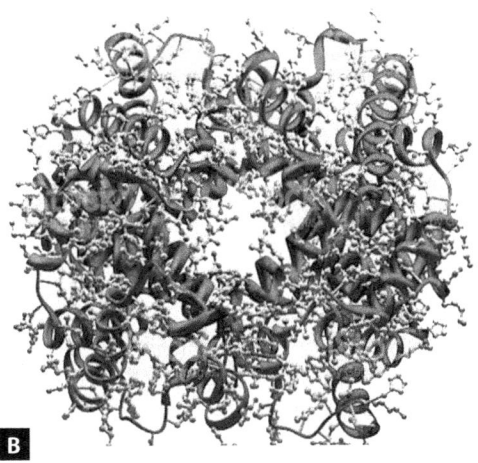

Figs. 1A and B: Structure of hemoglobin. (A) RBC; (B) Hemoglobin molecule.

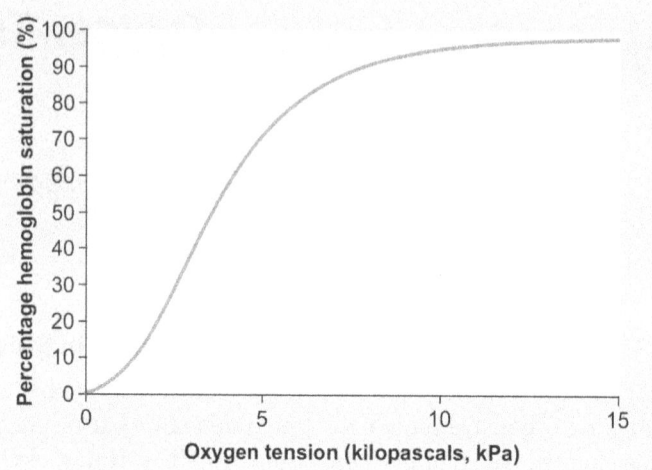

Fig. 2: Oxyhemoglobin dissociation curve (ODC).

of Hb. This relationship is best described by the sigmoid-shaped oxyhemoglobin dissociation curve (ODC) **(Fig. 2)**.

Oxyhemoglobin Dissociation Curve

- The curve is nonlinear and sigmoid.
- The Hb saturation with oxygen plateaus above 80 mm Hg but changes between 20 and 60 mm Hg.
- There are two forms of Hb: (1) Taut or tense (T), which has a low affinity for oxygen; and (2) Relaxed (R), which has a high affinity for oxygen. The taut form predominates in the tissues (high carbon dioxide, low pH environment) promoting oxygen release, whereas the relaxed form binds to oxygen more avidly in areas of high pH, low carbon dioxide tension, and high partial pressures of oxygen (such as in the alveoli).
- *Bohr effect:* Increase in the partial pressure of carbon dioxide in the blood or decrease in blood pH results in a lower affinity of Hb for oxygen, causing a shift of ODC to the right. It allows for enhanced unloading of oxygen in metabolically active peripheral tissues, such as exercising skeletal muscle.
- The primary factor determining whether oxygen is loaded or unloaded on to or from Hb is the partial pressure of oxygen.
- Carbon dioxide is returned to the lungs from the tissues as bicarbonate and carbamino Hb.
- *Haldane effect:* Deoxygenated blood has a greater ability to transport carbon dioxide when compared with oxygenated blood.
- The Bohr and Haldane effects promote oxygen binding and carbon dioxide release in the pulmonary capillaries with the reverse occurring in the tissues.
- *P50:* It is the partial pressure of oxygen at which Hb is 50% saturated (normal P50 is 27 mm Hg).
- *2,3-Diphosphoglycerate (2,3-DPG):* Also called 2,3-bisphosphoglycerate (BPG), it is produced in erythrocytes, which promotes Hb oxygen release.
- Inorganic phosphate is a substrate for the production of 2,3-DPG and thus capillary Hb oxygen release may be impaired, if hypophosphatemia is present and not corrected. In critical care, hypophosphatemia is seen in sepsis, refeeding syndrome,

postsurgical patients, diabetic ketoacidosis, acute liver injury, and during renal replacement therapy.

Table 1 summarizes the factors affecting ODC.

Oxygen Content

Oxygen content of arterial blood is the sum of the oxygen bound to Hb and the oxygen dissolved in plasma. It is the amount of oxygen in each 100 mL of blood and is calculated by the equation:

Oxygen delivery = cardiac output × arterial oxygen content

$$DO_2 = CO \times [1.39 \times Hb \times SaO_2 + (0.003 \times PaO_2)]$$

DO_2: Rate of oxygen delivery (mL/min)

CO: Cardiac output (L/min)

Oxygen-binding capacity of Hb: 1.39 mL/g

SaO_2: Hb oxygen saturation expressed as a fraction

Amount of dissolved oxygen in blood: 0.003 in 100 mL

Global oxygen delivery describes the amount of oxygen delivered to the tissues in each minute and is a product of the cardiac output and arterial oxygen content **(Table 2)**.
- *Stagnant anoxia:* Reduced cardiac output or regional blood flow
- *Anoxic anoxia:* Arterial hypoxemia

TABLE 1: Factors affecting oxyhemoglobin dissociation curve.

	LEFT($\downarrow$P50)	RIGHT ($\uparrow$P50)
Causes	$\uparrow$pH	$\downarrow$pH
	($\downarrow$H⁺)	($\uparrow$H⁺)
	$\downarrow$PaCO$_2$	$\uparrow$PaCO$_2$
	$\downarrow$2,3-DPG	$\uparrow$2,3-DPG
	$\downarrow$Temperature	$\uparrow$Temperature
Effect	Increased Hb oxygen affinity	Decreased Hb oxygen affinity
	Enhanced oxygen binding	Enhanced release of oxygen in the tissues
Others	Fetal Hb	Adult Hb
	Carbon monoxide poisoning	
	Methemoglobinemia	

(2,3-DPG: 2,3-diphosphoglycerate; PaCO$_2$: arterial carbon dioxide tension)

TABLE 2: Factors affecting oxygen delivery.

Type of hypoxia	[O$_2$]$_a$ (vol%)	[O$_2$]$_v$ (vol%)	CO (L/min)	VO$_2$ (mL/min)
Normoxia	20	15	5	250
Stagnant	Normal	$\downarrow$	$\downarrow\downarrow$	Normal
Hypoxic	$\downarrow\downarrow$	$\downarrow$	$\uparrow$	Normal
Anemic	$\downarrow\downarrow$	$\downarrow$	Normal or $\uparrow$	Normal
Histotoxic	Normal	$\uparrow$	Normal	$\downarrow\downarrow$

(CO: cardiac output; VO$_2$: oxygen consumption)

- *Anemic anoxia:* Reduced Hb
- *Cytopathic hypoxia:* Sepsis
- *Histotoxic hypoxia:* Cyanide poisoning

Oxygen Consumption

- Oxygen consumption (VO_2) is the amount of oxygen consumed by the tissues per minute.
- It can be calculated either through direct analysis of respiratory gases or indirectly, using Fick's principle, by measuring the oxygen content of mixed venous blood (i.e., blood in the pulmonary arteries), CvO_2, and using the equations:

$$CvO_2 = (1.31 \times Hb \times SvO_2 \times 0.01) + (0.0225 \times PvO_2)$$

$$VO_2 = CO \times (CaO_2 - CvO_2)$$

CaO_2 is arterial oxygen content.
- Factors that increase VO_2 include exercise, trauma, surgery, burns, inflammation, sepsis, pyrexia, shivering, pain, agitation, and physiotherapy (patients in critical care).

Factors that decrease VO_2 are sedation, analgesia, neuromuscular blocking agents, antipyretics, hypovolemia, shock states, mechanical ventilation, and hypothermia.

Oxygen Extraction Ratio

- Oxygen extraction ratio (OER) is the fraction of oxygen delivered via the cardiovascular system that is actually utilized by the tissues.
- It is the ratio of VO_2 to oxygen delivery:

  - $OER = \dfrac{VO_2}{DO_2}$ globally

  - $OER = \dfrac{CaO_2 - CvO_2}{CaO_2}$ or

  - $OER = \dfrac{O_2 in - O_2 out}{O_2 in}$ at the tissue level

- Under normal circumstances, 20–30% of the oxygen delivered to the tissues is utilized (an OER 0.2–0.3) and VO_2 is "supply-independent" and it is maintained. However, at a critical DO_2 (DO_2crit) of ~4 mL/kg/min in humans, the OER is maximal (OER 0.6–0.8) and VO_2 is said to become "supply-dependent."
- If DO_2 continues to decrease further below the DO_2crit, or if VO_2 increases, tissue hypoxia, anaerobic respiration, and lactate production begin secondary to an imbalance between ATP supply and demand.
- Pulmonary artery catheter-guided measurement of mixed venous blood saturation (SVO_2) or central venous oxygen saturation ($ScVO_2$) can be used to measure DO_2.

DIFFUSIVE OXYGEN TRANSPORT

- Henry's law states that the concentration of a gas within a liquid is proportional to its partial pressure within that liquid.
- *Fick's laws of diffusion:* Adolf Fick (1829–1901) derived two laws of diffusion in 1855. His first law states that at a steady state, particles move from an area of high concentration to an area of low concentration, the rate of which is proportional to the difference in their concentrations. Fick's second law describes how diffusion causes the concentration gradient to change with respect to time.
- Oxygen is released from Hb as RBCs flow through the capillaries and diffuses in mitochondria where it is utilized. Oxygen passes from the blood to tissues by diffusion.

  Krogh's cylinder model was developed to analyze oxygen transport to tissue. It is a simplified model of tissue surrounding a capillary.

The assumption of the model is that capillary is cylindrical with a constant radius and oxygen exchange happens between capillary and the surrounding cylindrical tissue. It also assumes that oxygen diffuses radially and oxygen tension is uniform. Hence, true VO_2 is underestimated. Various models have been described along with equations to explain oxygen transport across capillaries and arterioles and are beyond the scope of this chapter.

CLINICAL RELEVANCE

- *Cardiopulmonary exercise testing:* It is a tool to assess a patient's preoperative functional capacity before a major surgery. Anaerobic threshold is VO_2 where anaerobic metabolism starts; it can also be calculated.
- *Goal-directed hemodynamic therapy (GDT):* In GDT, blood flow and/or oxygen delivery (DO_2) is augmented through the use of supplemental oxygen and fluids (both crystalloids and colloids), inotropes, vasopressors, and vasodilators. A variety of physiological variables have been targeted including DO_2, cardiac index (CI), stroke volume (SV), and indexed systemic vascular resistance (SVRI).

ARTIFICIAL OXYGEN CARRIERS

Hemoglobin-based Oxygen Carriers

Hemoglobin-based oxygen carriers (HBOCs) are made from expired human blood or fresh bovine blood, which undergoes numerous modifications. Four types are cross-linked hemoglobins, cross-linked and polymerized hemoglobins, hemoglobins conjugated to macromolecules, and encapsulated hemoglobins. HBOC reacts with nitric oxide, leading to vasoconstriction and pressor effect within 15 minutes, and increases the oxygen-carrying capacity of blood and produces an oversupply of oxygen to the tissues, resulting in a compensatory autoregulatory vasoconstriction.

Perfluorocarbon Emulsions

Perfluorocarbon-based emulsions (PFCs) are mixtures of fluorocarbons and emulsifying agents. They are capable of delivering oxygen to the tissues passively and can carry an amount of oxygen proportional to the ambient PO_2 without having to rely on the RBCs. The half-life of PFCs is 2-4 hours and they are eliminated unmetabolized through the lungs after being taken up by the reticuloendothelial system (RES).

Maximal VO_2 is due to mitochondrial respiration. The site within the mitochondria at which oxygen is consumed is cytochrome *c* oxidase—the terminal electron acceptor in the electron transport chain. When NO levels at the mitochondria are high, VO_2 will be low; when NO levels are low, VO_2 will be high.

Our circle of life revolves around multiple complex cycles and transport mechanisms at the cellular level. The pandemic much emphasized the role of oxygen in our lives. We need to build up oxygen reserves for the future.

SUGGESTED READING

1. Dunn J-OC, Mythen MG, Grocott MP: Physiology of oxygen transport. BJA Educ. 2016;16(10):341-8.
2. Hsia CCW, Respiratory function of hemoglobin. N Engl J Med. 1998;338(4):239-48.
3. Pittman RN. Oxygen transport. Regulation of Tissue Oxygenation. San Rafael: Morgan & Claypool Life Sciences; 2011.

Oxyhemoglobin Dissociation Curve

CHAPTER 12

Srinivas Samavedam, Shabeer Ahmed Khan

INTRODUCTION

Oxygen is carried in the body mainly in the bound state, and a minor portion of it is carried in a dissolved form in the blood plasma. About 98% of oxygen is carried in a protein-bound state to hemoglobin (Hb), which is approximately 197 mL/L. Only 2% of oxygen is carried in a dissolved state in the plasma. In a healthy adult, each 100 mL of blood contains 15 g of Hb. Each gram of Hb can carry 1.34 mL of oxygen. Therefore, each 100 mL of blood containing 15 g of Hb can carry approximately 20 mL of oxygen when Hb is 100% saturated. Under normal physiological conditions, when systemic arterial blood is 97% saturated, each 100 mL of blood contains 19.4 mL of oxygen. However, at the tissue capillary level, the amount is reduced to 14.4 mL of oxygen per 100 mL of blood. So, each 100 mL of blood flowing from the lungs to tissue capillaries transports approximately 5 mL of blood. According to Henry's Law, the dissolved fraction is proportional to the atmospheric pressure of oxygen in blood (PO_2), but the solubility of oxygen is so low that only 3 mL of oxygen per 1 L of blood is dissolved at atmospheric oxygen tension. The oxygen content of arterial blood is approximately 20 g/dL, the oxygen content of venous blood is 15 g/dL, and dissolved oxygen contributes 0.1 g/dL in each case (but is continuously replenished from the Hb bound pool).

MECHANISM

Each Hb molecule contains a nonprotein moiety called heme and a protein called globin. Each Hb molecule contains four subunits: two α subunits and two β subunits. Each α and β subunit carries a separate heme group and globin chain. The heme portion of the Hb contains a ferrous (Fe^{2+}) of iron atom at its core that can bind to one oxygen molecule. So, each Hb tetramer can carry four oxygen molecules. Hb exists in two states—the T state (deoxygenated or tense) state and the oxygenated R (relaxed) state. The two states differ in their ability to bind to oxygen. The T state requires a higher PO_2 to bind an oxygen atom, like that found in the oxygen-rich pulmonary capillary beds. Most of the Hb exists in the T state in an unbound state and the binding of oxygen occurs with low affinity. The binding of each oxygen molecule induces conformational changes in other subunits toward the R state, thereby facilitating the binding of subsequent oxygen molecules. The interaction between Hb subunits is called *cooperativity*. The binding of the first oxygen molecule facilitates the binding of second, third, and fourth oxygen molecules, which is called positive cooperativity. Throughout the circulation, there is a continuum between the T state and the R state, in which unloading occurs.

OXYHEMOGLOBIN DISSOCIATION CURVE

Relationship between the partial pressure of oxygen plotted on the x-axis and the percentage saturation of Hb on the y-axis is called oxyhemoglobin dissociation curve (ODC). The ODC is a sigmoid-shaped curve, which describes the binding of oxygen to Hb at various levels **(Fig. 1)**. At the pulmonary capillary level, where the oxygen tension is high, the ODC plateaus. At the tissue level, where the oxygen tension is low, there will be release of oxygen from Hb, represented by the steeper portion of the oxyhemoglobin curve. 1 g of Hb can carry 1.34 mL of oxygen. The ODC shows that as the partial pressure of oxygen increases, the percentage of Hb bound to oxygen increases, which is called percentage saturation of Hb. The partial pressure of oxygen at which Hb is 50% saturated is called P50. The P50 of ODC is 26 mm Hg. The systemic arterial blood when it is 97% saturated has a partial pressure of oxygen in arterial blood (PaO_2) of 95 mm Hg, the blood returning to lungs has a partial pressure of oxygen in mixed venous blood (PvO_2) of 40 mm Hg, and the saturation averages 70–75%.

The sigmoid shape of the curve is significant for three reasons:
1. When Hb >92% saturated, a modest fall in PaO_2 will only have little effect on the oxygen content.
2. There will not be any significant change in the arterial content on increasing the PaO_2 beyond normal.
3. At the steeper portion of the curve (at saturation <90%), even a slight increase or decrease in PaO_2 can cause a significant increase or decrease in the oxygen content respectively.

When oxygen is loaded or unloaded from Hb, it is determined by the prevailing PO_2. There is a range over which loading (association) and unloading (dissociation) take place. The significance of this range is that loading takes place over a wide range of PO_2. As a result, over 90% saturations can be achieved from a PO_2 as low as 60 mm Hg. Similarly, at the tissue level, where unloading

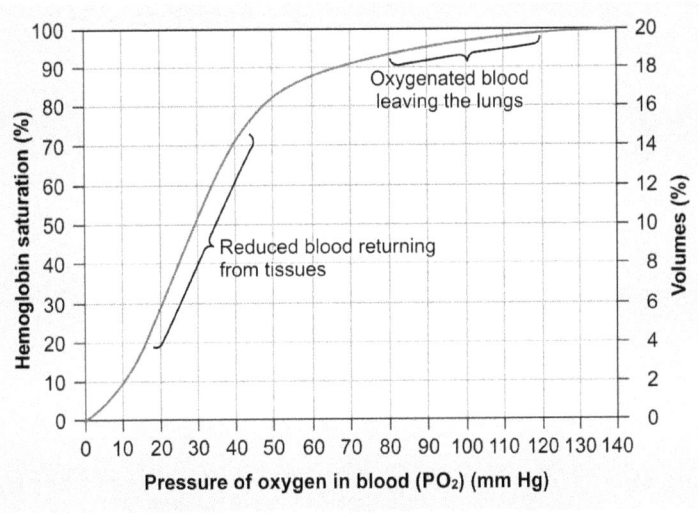

Fig. 1: Oxyhemoglobin dissociation curve.

is required, a relatively small decrease in PO_2 results in large unloading of oxygen.

Utilization Coefficient

Utilization coefficient is the percentage of blood that gives up oxygen as it passes through a tissue. Normally, it is 25%. During exercise, it is increased to 75–85% or even higher.

Factors Affecting the Oxyhemoglobin Dissociation Curve

A shift of the curve to the right decreases the affinity of Hb for oxygen and facilitates the release of oxygen to tissues. A leftward shift of the curve increases the tendency of Hb to take up oxygen. The amount by which the curve is shifted may be expressed by P50 oxygen. The P50 of adult Hb is 26.5 mm Hg (3.5 kPa) (Table 1).

pH and Bohr Effect

Acidity causes rightward shift of the dissociation curve, while alkalinity shifts the curve to the left. The increase in H^+ facilitates a stabilization of Hb in the T state, leading to unloading and rightward shift of ODC. At the tissue level, glucose and oxygen are metabolized into carbon dioxide and organic acids, causing reduced affinity of Hb to oxygen and helps in delivery of oxygen to tissues (Fig. 2).

The Bohr effect is a phenomenon first described in 1904 by a Danish physiologist, Christian Bohr. It is the shift of the ODC to

TABLE 1: Factors affecting the oxyhemoglobin dissociation curve.

Factors causing right shift of ODC	Factors causing left shift of ODC
Decrease in pH	Increase in pH
Increase in CO_2	Decrease in CO_2
Exercise	Increase in 2,3-DPG
Increase in 2,3-DPG	Hypothermia
Hyperthermia	

(2,3-DPG: 2,3-diphosphoglycerate; ODC: oxyhemoglobin dissociation curve)

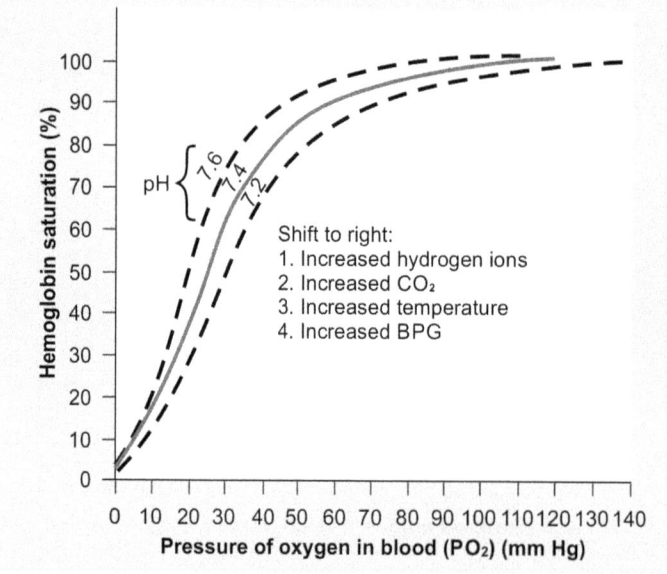

Fig. 2: Factors causing right shift of oxyhemoglobin dissociation curve.
(BPG: 2,3-biphosphoglycerate)

the right, as the partial pressure of carbon dioxide increases. In other words, the oxygen-binding affinity of Hb is inversely related to the concentration of carbon dioxide. As the blood passes through the tissues, carbon dioxide diffuses from tissue into the blood, resulting in an increase in the partial pressure of carbon dioxide (PCO_2) in blood levels. Majority of carbon dioxide is carried in a bicarbonate buffer system. Inside the red cells, the carbon dioxide is converted to carbonic acid in the presence of enzyme carbonic anhydrase, which further dissociates into HCO_3^- and H^+.

Carbon Dioxide

Increase in carbon dioxide concentrations causes rightward shift of the curve by two ways: (1) the Bohr effect and (2) the increase in carbamino compounds, leading to increased production and dissociation of carbonic acid, thereby causing a fall in blood pH and facilitating the unloading of oxygen from Hb.

2,3-Diphosphoglycerate Levels

2,3-diphosphoglycerate (2,3-DPG) is a metabolically important phosphate compound present in blood. It is produced in red blood cells as an intermediate product of glycolysis. An increase in 2,3-DPG levels causes a rightward shift of ODC and a decrease in 2,3-DPG shifts the curve to the left. At high altitude, hyperventilation causes a fall in PCO_2 and hydrogen loss, causing a leftward shift of ODC. This leads to an increase in the red cell production of 2,3-DPG, leading to a rightward shift of the curve, enabling unloading of oxygen from Hb as an important compensatory mechanism. So, the DPG mechanism is an important adaptation to hypoxia caused by poor blood flow in the tissues.

Exercise

Exercise causes release of large amounts of carbon dioxide along with other acids, which increases the H^+ concentration, leading to a fall in pH. Exercise causes an increase in the temperature of the muscle by 2–3°C, which facilitates oxygen delivery to the muscle fibers.

Fetal Hemoglobin

Fetal Hb consists of two α and two γ subunits. Compared to adult Hb, it has a significantly higher affinity for oxygen and causes a leftward shift of ODC at the level of placenta. 2,3-DPG interacts more readily with adult Hb, inducing oxygen unloading, and it allows the fetus to extract more oxygen from maternal circulation. The fetal Hb remains unaffected by 2,3-DPG and binds to oxygen firmly. Following birth, it is almost completely replaced by adult Hb at 6 months after birth.

Carbon Monoxide

Carbon monoxide diffuses rapidly across the pulmonary capillary membrane and binds to iron moiety of heme. The affinity of carbon monoxide to Hb is 200–250 times higher

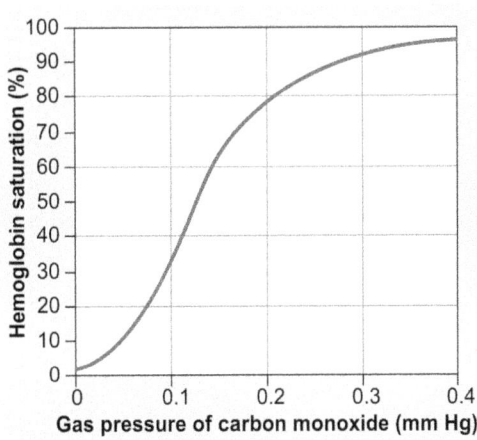

Fig. 3: Carbon monoxide–hemoglobin dissociation curve.

compared to oxygen. In the presence of carbon monoxide, oxygen binding is impaired and it binds with Hb, displacing oxygen and causing a leftward shift of ODC. Once carbonmonoxy binds to the heme moiety of Hb, an allosteric change diminishes the ability of other three oxygen-binding sites to off-load oxygen to peripheral tissues and impairs tissue-oxygen delivery **(Fig. 3)**.

SUGGESTED READING

1. Goldberg S, Heitner S, Mimouni F, Joseph L, Bromiker R, Picard E. The influence of reducing fever on blood oxygen saturation in children. Eur J Pediatr. 2018;177(1):95-9.
2. Hall, J. E. (2016). Guyton and Hall Textbook of Medical Physiology, 14th edition. Philadelphia, PA: Elsevier.
3. Mateják M, Kulhánek T, Matoušek S. Adair-based hemoglobin equilibrium with oxygen, carbon dioxide and hydrogen ion activity. Scand J Clin Lab Invest. 2015;75(2):113-20.
4. Patel S, Jose A, Mohiuddin SS. Physiology, Oxygen Transport and Carbon Dioxide Dissociation Curve. In: StatPearls [online]. StatPearls Publishing; Treasure Island (FL): 2021.
5. Svedenkrans J, Stoecklin B, Jones JG, Doherty DA, Pillow JJ. Physiology and predictors of impaired gas exchange in infants with bronchopulmonary dysplasia. Am J Respir Crit Care Med. 2019;200(4):471-80.

Diffusion of Oxygen and its Applied Physiology

CHAPTER

Srinivas Samavedam, Kiran Raghavendra Asrnanna

INTRODUCTION

Oxygen diffuses from the alveoli to pulmonary capillaries due to presence of a gradient driven between the partial pressure of oxygen in the alveoli and the pulmonary capillaries. Gas exchange portions of the lung exist distal to terminal bronchioles, and both oxygen and carbon dioxide exchange occurs at the alveolar level. Given the efficiency of alveolar gas diffusion, pulmonary end capillary blood/gas partial pressure exactly reflects alveolar gas composition. All gas transport across the pulmonary capillaries occurs through passive diffusion down a concentration gradient.

The diffusion equilibrium is mostly achieved for oxygen during the normal pulmonary capillary transit time in the resting subject, the uptake of oxygen is *limited by pulmonary blood flow* and not by diffusing capacity. However, when exercising at reduced barometric pressure or gas mixture deficient in oxygen, *the diffusing capacity becomes important* and may limit oxygen uptake.

Diffusion was described by Fick's law of diffusion or Brownian motion of diffusing particles.

FICK'S LAW OF DIFFUSION

Fick's law of diffusion states that at a steady state, particles move from an area of higher concentration to an area of lower concentration, and the rate is proportional to the difference in their concentrations.

The rate of diffusion of gas:

$$\text{FLUX} = \frac{DA\,(C1-C2)}{T}$$

where D is diffusion constant for a specific gas at a specified temperature and A is the surface area of gas exchange. The surface area is the area that is capable of exchanging gas on the alveolar and capillary sides.

$C1-C2$ is the concentration gradient of the gas across the membrane.

The larger the PO_2 difference between the alveolus and capillary, the greater the rate of diffusion. Thus, a much greater alveolar-capillary PO_2 gradient is required to maintain oxygen transport. The mixed venous blood entering the pulmonary capillary has a PO_2 of 40 mm Hg, and the alveolar PO_2 is approximately 100 mm Hg, therefore the pressure gradient is 60 mm Hg. If the mixed venous PO_2 is lower than normal, the pressure gradient increases and partially compensates toward achieving equilibrium with alveolar O_2.

When the blood flows through the capillary, it takes up oxygen and delivers carbon dioxide, but because oxygen partial pressure builds up in the capillary bed, the diffusion rate slows down and becomes zero when the pressure is equilibrated across the alveolar–capillary wall.

T is the capillary wall thickness. Thickened alveolar–capillary membrane also decreases the diffusion, because the longer the diffusion distance, the lower is the diffusion capacity.

Thus,
- The rate of diffusion of a gas through a tissue slice is proportional to the area but inversely proportional to the thickness.
- Diffusion rate is proportional to the partial pressure difference.
- Diffusion rate is proportional to the solubility of the gas in the tissue, but inversely proportional to the square root of the molecular weight.

$$D \propto \frac{\text{Solubility}}{\sqrt{MW}}$$

where D is the diffusion, solubility is the gas solubility, and MW is the molecular weight of the gas.

The larger the molecule, the slower the diffusion. The molecular weight of oxygen is 32, molecular weight of carbon dioxide is 44, but the carbon dioxide transport across the alveolar membrane is *twenty times greater* than that of oxygen under the same partial pressure, because the solubility of carbon dioxide in water is 20 times greater than the solubility of oxygen.

$$\text{Diffusing capacity} = \frac{\text{Net rate of gas transfer}}{\text{Partial pressure gradient}}$$

The biological unit of diffusing capacity is mL/min/mm Hg.

Factors that influence the diffusional conductance of gas include the thickness of blood, gas barrier, alveolar-capillary surface area, the solubility of a gas in blood, gas barrier and molecular weight of the gas.

Additional factors include:
- *Capillary transit time:* The transit time of blood in alveolar capillaries (called pulmonary transit time) is normally 0.75–1 second. It reflects the ratio of microcirculatory blood volume to blood flow. If there is a disease affecting the alveolar-capillary membrane, even a normal capillary transit time may be insufficient for adequate gas diffusion.

The reaction rate of O_2 is fast, but because so little time is available in the capillary, this rate can become a limiting factor. The resistance to the uptake of O_2 attributable to reaction rate is probably about the same as that due to diffusion across the blood–gas barrier. In this way, the separate contributions of the diffusion properties of the blood–gas barrier and the volume of capillary blood can be derived.

At rest, equilibrium is reached within 25–30% of the capillary length, and almost no gas transfer occurs in the remaining capillary. During exercise and stress, blood flow through the capillary is faster, and a longer capillary distance is required before equilibrium is reached.
- *Protein-gas binding rate:* The binding of hemoglobin and O_2 has a finite rate, which is faster than the diffusion rate.
- *The capacity of hemoglobin to carry the gas:* Most of the O_2 that dissolves in the plasma diffuses into the red cell and binds to hemoglobin. The hemoglobin-bound with O_2 creates no pressure in the plasma, and thus it allows much more oxygen to diffuse across the membranes before a pressure equilibration is reached.

Measurement of Diffusion Capacity

A single breath test is a frequently used test in which a single inspiration of a dilute carbon monoxide is made to inspire and the rate of disappearance of carbon monoxide from the alveolar gas during a 10-second breath-hold is calculated. The concentrations of inspired and expired carbon monoxide are measured with an infrared analyzer.

The normal value of the diffusing capacity for carbon monoxide at rest is about

25 mL/min or mm/Hg, and it increases to two or three times this value during exercise because of the recruitment and distension of pulmonary capillaries.

ALVEOLAR–ARTERIAL GRADIENT

The alveolar-arterial gradient, or the A-a gradient, estimates the difference between the oxygen concentration in the alveoli and arterial system. The A-a gradient helps in narrowing the differential diagnosis for hypoxemia.

$$\text{A-a gradient} = P_AO_2 - P_aO_2$$

P_AO_2 represents the alveolar oxygen pressure and P_aO_2 represents arterial oxygen pressure. The partial pressure of oxygen (P_aO_2) can be directly assessed with an arterial blood gas (ABG). The partial pressure of oxygen in the alveolus (P_AO_2) is not easily measured directly; instead, it is estimated by using the alveolar gas equation:

$$P_AO_2 = (P_{atm} - P_{H_2O}) F_iO_2 - P_aCO_2/RQ$$

In a healthy adult, the A-a gradient would be negligible: Oxygen would diffuse and equalize across the capillary membrane, and the pressure difference in the arterial system and alveoli would be minimal.

The A-a gradient changes with the patient's age. The expected A-a gradient can be estimated with the following equation:

$$\text{A-a gradient} = (\text{Age} + 10)/4$$

The calculated value for a patient's A-a gradient can be used to assess if the hypoxia is due to the dysfunction of the alveolar-capillary unit. Hypoxemia in a patient due to hypoventilation [central nervous system (CNS) depression, kyphoscoliosis, neuromuscular weakness] will have an A-a gradient within normal limits. Hypoxemic patients with a parenchymal diseases like pneumonia will have an inappropriately elevated A-a gradient. An elevated A-a gradient indicates that the partial pressure of O_2 is higher in the alveoli than in arterial blood, indicating a V/Q mismatch.

Elevated A-a gradient can also be present due to:
- *Dead space ventilation:* Pneumonia, chronic obstructive pulmonary disease (COPD), pulmonary embolism
- *Left-to-right shunt:* Acute respiratory distress syndrome (ARDS), pulmonary edema
- *Alveolar hypoventilation:* Pulmonary fibrosis, interstitial lung disease

FACTORS THAT AFFECT THE DIFFUSION OF GAS ACROSS THE ALVEOLAR MEMBRANE

- In lung diseases, failure of diffusional equilibration is rarely seen. It appears to be consistently measured only in patients with interstitial lung diseases, and is seen most often when they exercise. Only in severe cases of interstitial lung disease when lung function is at 50% of normal or less.
- When alveolar-capillary membrane is thin, the diffusion is faster, conditions which cause thickening of the barrier, impair the diffusion.
- The larger the surface area of the alveolar-capillary membrane, the faster the rate of diffusion. Numerous alveoli help in gas exchange. Some diseases such as emphysema lead to the destruction of alveolar architecture, which causes the formation of bullae. This reduces the surface area available for diffusion, thereby decreasing the rate of diffusion.
- If the end-capillary partial pressure of the gas being exchanged is not equal to its alveolar value, in any homogeneous lung region, there can be diffusion limitations.

- Chronic heart failure with pulmonary edema causes pulmonary capillary congestion increasing the length of the diffusion pathway for oxygen through plasma, interstitial edema increasing the thickness of the membrane, or raised capillary pressure damaging the endothelial and epithelial cells leading to the proliferation of type II alveolar cells and thickening of the membrane.
- Anemia reduces the diffusion capacity, whereas polycythemia increases the diffusion capacity.
- Stature influences diffusion capacity directly due to the relationship between height and lung volume.
- Diffusion capacity is substantially increased when the subject is supine rather than standing or sitting.
- Diffusion capacity decreases with increasing age.
- Women generally have reduced diffusional capacity in comparison to men.

SUGGESTED READING

1. Leach RM, Treacher DF. The pulmonary physician in critical care * 2: oxygen delivery and consumption in the critically ill. Thorax. 2002;57(2):170-7.
2. Nunn JF. Nunn's Applied Respiratory Physiology, 4th edition. Oxford: Butterworth-Heinemann; 1993.
3. Thomas C, Lumb AB. Physiology of haemoglobin. Contin Educ Anaesth Crit Care Pain. 2012;12:251-6.
4. West JB. Respiratory physiology: The Essentials, 7th edition. London: Lippincott Williams & Wilkins; 2004.

CHAPTER 14

Pulse Oximetry: Understanding and Limitations

Kanwalpreet Sodhi, Manender Kumar

INTRODUCTION

Pulse oximetry, termed as "the fifth vital sign", is a noninvasive method of determining oxygen saturation (SaO_2) of arterial blood. It provides continuous display of the oxygenation by a rapid and accurate method making it the standard of care in operation theatres, recovery rooms, intensive care units, wards as well as during transport of patients in and out of the hospitals. Pulse oximetry can help in early detection of hypoxemia before other manifestations such as cyanosis or change in heart rate, thereby allowing early treatment much before the tissue damage and other possible complications. Assessment of oxygenation status has been included by the American Society of Anesthesiology (ASA), World Federation of Societies of Anesthesiologist, World Health Organization (WHO), and American Association of Nurse Anesthetists as the minimum monitoring standard for intraoperative and postoperative monitoring. The use of pulse oximetry is a part of WHO safe surgery checklist. In 2005, ASA added the requirement of variable pulse pitch tone making auditory detection of low SpO_2 values possible, even without looking at the monitor. Indian Society of Anesthesiologists has included pulse oximetry as the desirable standard to monitor oxygenation during anesthesia.

PRINCIPLE

Adult blood contains five types of hemoglobin (Hb): (1) oxyhemoglobin (O_2Hb), (2) deoxyhemoglobin (deO_2Hb), (3) carboxyhemoglobin (COHb), (4) methemoglobin (MetHb), and (5) sulfhemoglobin (SulfHb). Fractional SaO_2 (%HbO_2) is calculated as amount of O_2Hb as fraction of total amount of Hb, whether functional or not. Functional SaO_2 refers to ratio of O_2Hb to only functional hemoglobins, i.e., O_2Hb and deO_2Hb.

$$\%HbO_2 = \frac{O_2Hb}{O_2Hb + deO_2Hb + CoHb + MetHb + SHb} \times 100\%$$

$$SaO_2 = \frac{O_2Hb}{O_2Hb + deO_2Hb} \times 100\%$$

Recognition of two facts is very important in understanding the principle of pulse oximetry:
1. It has to distinguish between O_2Hb from deO_2Hb.
2. It has to calculate the SpO_2 from only the pulsatile arterial component of the blood.

Pulse oximetry combines the spectrophotometry and plethysmography technology. Spectrophotometry involves calculating the amount of O_2Hb and deO_2Hb by their differential absorption of different frequencies of light. Pulse oximetry principle makes use of *Beer–Lambart law* that relates the transmission of light through a solution to the concentration of the solute in the solution. Thus the concentration of the solute in a solution can be known by amount of light of a particular wavelength absorbed and transmitted through the solution. For calculating the concentrations of multiple solutes, lights of different wavelengths, at least equal to number of solutes have to be used. Commonly used pulse oximeters use lights of two frequencies that readily penetrate the tissues: red light of frequency 660 nm and infrared light of frequency 940 nm. These two frequency lights are differentially absorbed by O_2Hb and deO_2Hb. O_2Hb absorbs more light in 940 nm band than deO_2Hb and deO_2Hb absorbs more light than O_2Hb in 660 nm band. The pulse oximeter probe emits these two lights: red light at 660 nm and infrared light at 940 nm, by a pair of light emitting diodes (LEDs) present in one arm of probe. A photodetector is present usually on the opposite side of probe that detects the amounts of transmitted lights. The proportion of O_2Hb is calculated by relative absorbance and transmission of the two lights.

The pulse oximeter calculates the SaO_2 of only arterial blood by taking advantage of pulsatile nature of arterial blood (Plethysmography), the reason term SpO_2 (oxygen saturation obtained from the pulse) is used. The amount of red and infrared lights absorbed fluctuates with the cardiac cycle, as the arterial blood volume increases during systole, and decreases during diastole; in contrast, the blood volume in the veins and capillaries as well as the volumes of skin, fat, bone, etc., remain relatively constant. So the absorption of light by the tissue has two components: steady direct current (DC) component and pulsatile alternating current (AC) component (taken from DC and AC in physics) **(Fig. 1)**. To detect these AC and DC components, pulse oximeter LEDs operate in sequence at a rate of several hundred times per second. The LEDs are turned on and off

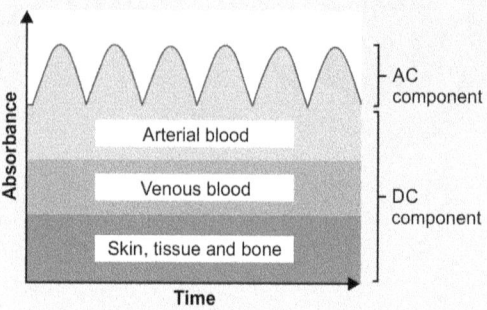

Fig. 1: Schematic representation of absorbance of light by different body components.

in sequence, enabling the photodetector to measure the transmission of each light **(Fig. 2)**. When both LEDs are turned off, photodetector measures the ambient light and subtracts it from the signals received in rest of the cycle. From the proportions of light absorbed by each component at the two frequencies, pulse-added absorbance (R) is calculated by the following formula:

$$R = \frac{AC660/DC660}{AC940/DC940}$$

where AC660, AC940, DC660, and DC940 represent AC and DC components of 660 nm and 940 nm wavelengths, respectively. This ratio R is subsequently analyzed by mathematical algorithms internal to each microprocessor in the pulse oximeter. These algorithms are developed by the manufacturers by breathing of hypoxic gas mixtures by the healthy volunteers to get SaO_2 values 70–100%. Pulse oximeter readings below 70% are not considered reliable because those values are calculated by extrapolation from the values recorded in the microprocessor.

In the newer designs, multiple wavelengths of light (more than seven) have been introduced which enables the measurement of Hb, oxygen content, and detection of other types of hemoglobins like COHb and MetHb, etc.

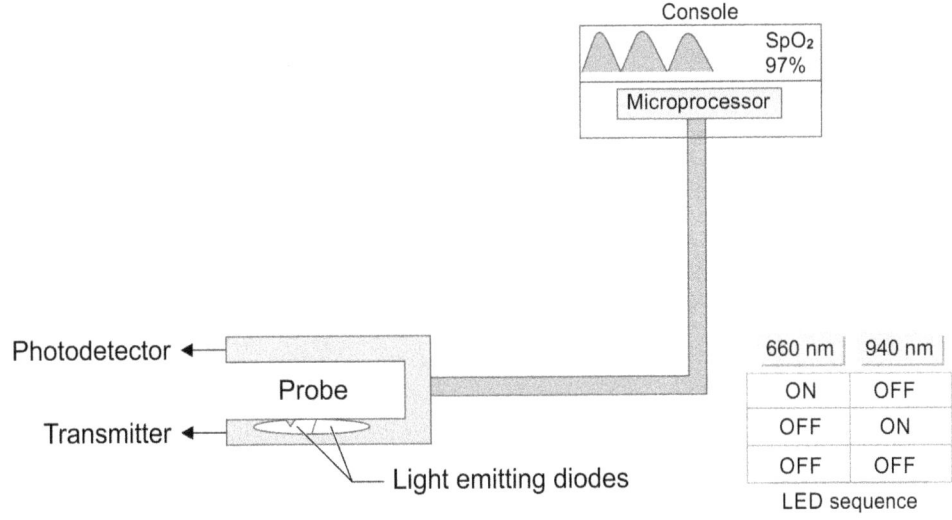

Fig. 2: Schematic representation showing working principle of pulse oximeter.

TABLE 1: SpO$_2$ probe positioning.	
Transmission oximetry probes usually placed on the fingers, toes, hands, feet, nose, ear, tongue, and cheek	Reflectance oximetry probes placed on esophagus, scalp, and forehead

COMPONENTS OF PULSE OXIMETER

The probe is the part that comes in direct contact with the patient. It consists of LEDs and the photodetector. Most probes are based on *transmission oximetry*, in which LEDs and photodetector are present on opposite side of each other and light is actually transmitted from the tissues. In others, *reflectance oximetry* is used which determine SpO$_2$ by the light that is reflected back (scattered). In this type, both the emitters and photodetector are on same side of the probe **(Table 1)**.

Both reusable and single-use probes are available with varying advantages **(Table 2)**.

The probe is connected to the console by the cable. Cables from one manufacturer cannot be used into the others, although they may fit into each other.

TABLE 2: Comparison of reusable and disposable probes.	
Reusable probe	**Disposable or single use self-adhesive probe**
Can be applied rapidly	More secure placement
Easy to use in conditions of low-amplitude waveforms	Can be used when there is excessive patient movement
Cost-effective	Potentially lesser risk of nosocomial infections
	Allows monitoring of sites other than acral regions which are vulnerable to vasoconstriction e.g. scalp, forehead, nose etc.

Console is the part where data is analyzed using stored algorithms by the microprocessors. They can be standalone monitors or a part of multiparameter monitor. The SpO$_2$ value is shown with or without signal strength or plethysmographic waveform. Most pulse oximeters provide audible tone with variable pitch that change according to change in saturation. Nowadays handy, portable pulse oximeters are widely used that show heart rate, SpO$_2$, and plethysmographic waveform in the probe itself.

APPLICATIONS OF PULSE OXIMETRY

Pulse oximeter is a rapid, noninvasive, and bedside monitor for critically ill patients. The major advantages of pulse oximetry are enumerated in **Box 1**. It is a versatile parameter with numerous clinical applications:

- *Monitoring oxygenation:*
  - One of the very important tools to monitor oxygenation during anesthesia, in the recovery room, and diagnose hypoxia in wards and intensive care units.
  - As a tool to confirm tracheal tube placement when end-tidal CO$_2$ is not available. If the SpO$_2$ rises after intubation and ventilation, correct endotracheal tube placement is likely.
  - Pulse oximeter is a useful transport monitor to detect desaturation events.
- *Monitoring peripheral circulation:* When vascular supply to the limb may get compromised as may occur with limb in dependent position, fractures, etc., [Can be used in Modified Allen's test to check adequacy of collateral circulation in hand through palmar arterial arch (Barbeau Test)].
- *Monitoring systolic blood pressure:* By putting the blood-pressure cuff and pulse oximeter probe on the same limb, the cuff can be inflated till the plethysmographic waveform disappears or the cuff can be overinflated and deflated slowly and recording the blood pressure at the point when the waveform reappears.
- *Detecting Hyperoxemia:* Pulse oximetry can help *detecting hyperoxemia* that is detrimental in premature neonates, causing retinopathy and oxygen toxicity.
- *Detecting fluid responsiveness:* Since absorption of light is proportional to the changes in blood volume, changes calculated from plethysmographic waveform [pleth variability index (PVI)] is a reliable indicator of fluid responsiveness in perioperative period and in critically ill patients. A cutoff of PVI >14% indicates fluid responsiveness (normal PVI 9–13%) (**Fig. 3**).

DISADVANTAGES AND LIMITATIONS

Pulse oximetry has some fallacies in its clinical application due to unreliable SpO$_2$ readings (**Box 2**).

> **BOX 1:** Advantages of pulse oximetry.
>
> - Accurate and accuracy does not change over time; good correlation has been shown with blood gas analysis pO$_2$ values till SpO$_2$ of 70%
> - Accurate even in dysrhythmias, provided the SpO$_2$ is stable and waveform is of reasonable amplitude
> - Noninvasive and has faster response time than transcutaneous measurements
> - Application of probe is easy and fast
> - Perfusion can be indicated by pulse signal strength
> - Detection of hypoxemia is easier with variable pitch of pulse tone without even looking at the monitor

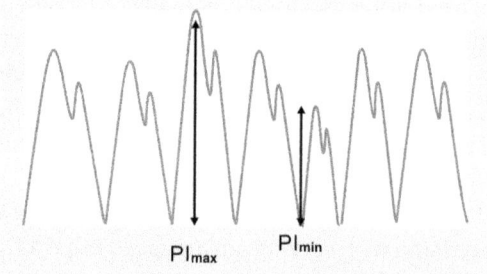

PVI = [(PI$_{max}$ − PI$_{min}$)/PI$_{max}$] × 100%

Fig. 3: Pleth variability index (PVI). (PI: perfusion index)

> **BOX 2:** Limitations of pulse oximetry due to unreliable SpO_2 readings.
>
> *Falsely low SpO_2*
> - Motion artifacts/excessive movement
> - Venous pulsations
> - *Dark nail polish:* Blue and green produce greater decreases than purple and red; black produces an intermediate decrease
>
> *Falsely normal or higher SpO_2*
> - Vaso-occlusive crisis in sickle cell anemia
> - Carbon monoxide (CO) poisoning
> - Carboxyhemoglobinemia
> - Severe anemia with severe hypoxemia
> - Any nail paint color other than blue/black
> - Intravenous pigmented dyes
>
> *Unpredictable SpO_2 (falsely low or high SpO_2)*
> - Sepsis and septic shock
> - Poor probe positioning
> - Methemoglobinemia
> - Sulfhemoglobinemia
> - Inherited hemoglobinopathies
>
> *Intermittent dropouts or inability to read SpO_2*
> - Poor perfusion
> - Hypovolemia
> - Severe vasoconstriction/excessive vasopressor use

- Pulse oximetry gives information only about saturation of circulating Hb. It does not give any information about tissue oxygenation.
- Accuracy is limited for SaO_2 values <70%.
- *Lag time:* There can be significant lag time between change in alveolar oxygen tension and corresponding pulse oximeter reading. This can be related to position of probe. More centrally placed probes detect desaturation earlier. It can also be due to poor perfusion as in cold extremities, peripheral vasoconstriction, venous obstruction, etc.
- Pulse oximeters may not work properly in presence of *dysrhythmias*. Also in patients on intra-aortic balloon pump, there can be double or triple peaked arterial and plethysmographic waveform leading on to inconsistent SpO_2 values.
- Presence of *venous pulsations* (as in severe tricuspid regurgitation, tight placement of adhesive probes, hyperemia of the limb, probe placement in dependent position, e.g., at forehead during Trendelenburg position), detection of venous O_2Hb may artifactually lower the arterial SpO_2 values.
- *Inaccuracies with presence of other Hb types:*
  - MetHb: Normally <1% of total Hb, metHb is an oxidation product of Hb that reversibly binds O_2 and impairs tissue oxygen delivery. MetHb absorbs significant amount of light at both 660 nm and 940 nm frequencies. It leads to absorbance ratio of 1, which corresponds to SpO_2 values close to 85. Thus in presence of methemoglobinemia (congenital or acquired), SpO_2 value will be 80–85% irrespective of SaO_2 values.
  - COHb: It is formed when carbon monoxide (CO) binds with Hb as in cases of CO poisoning. At 660 nm wavelength, COHb absorbs light in the same manner as of O_2Hb, but it absorbs virtually no light at 940 nm frequency. This leads to falsely elevated SpO_2 values compared with SaO_2 values.
  - SulfHb: It absorbs more light at both the frequencies leading to fixed SpO_2 values of 85% in cases of severe sulfhemoglobinemia.
  - Fetal hemoglobin (HbF): It does not significantly alter SpO_2 values.
  - Hemoglobin S: In sickle cell disease, many studies have found SpO_2 values to be accurate, but some studies suggest that SpO_2 values may overestimate SaO_2 especially during vaso-occlusive

crisis. Also heme metabolism may lead to increased COHb values.
- Congenital variants of hemoglobin: Hb Canebiere, Hb Rothschild, and Hb Bassett have lesser affinity to O_2. So changes in SpO_2 reflect changes in SaO_2. Other variants like Hb Lansing, Hb Koln, Hb Bonn, Hb Cheverly, and Hb Hammersmith absorb light similar to deO_2Hb resulting in lower SpO_2 values.
- Thus, whenever conflicting results are found in SpO_2 values and blood gas analysis, hemoglobinopathies should be suspected and confirmation should be done by co-oximetry and other additional tests.
- *Anemia:* Anemia usually has little or no impact on SpO_2 in presence of normal SaO_2. However in presence of hypoxia, SpO_2 readings may underestimate SaO_2.
- Severe *hyperbilirubinemia* (30 mg/dL or more) caused by hemolysis or liver disease can lead to artifactual increase in COHb and MetHb, but SpO_2 values are generally unaffected.
- *Sepsis and septic shock:* There are conflicting results on how SpO_2 get biased in septic shock. Based upon the extent of vasopressor use, fluid resuscitation, cardiac dysfunction, or associated comorbid conditions, the SpO_2 may be spuriously affected in any direction.
- *Intravenous dyes:* The administration of intravenous dyes may transiently lead to inaccurate SpO_2 readings. Methylene blue can decrease SpO_2 due to its peak absorption at 668 nm. Indigo carmine and indocyanine green also artificially decrease SpO_2 values. Isosulfan blue can cause SpO_2 reduction at prolonged doses.
- *Nail polish:* Although all nail colors can reduce calculated SpO_2 values, shades of purple, dark blue, black, and green having more effect. In such cases, the probe can be positioned side to side on the finger rather than on nail. Synthetic acrylic nails can also cause difficulty in detection of SpO_2.
- *Skin pigmentation* has usually no effect on SpO_2 values.
- *Ambient light* generally does not alter SpO_2 values but *flickering lights* with frequencies similar to LEDs, operating room lights, infrared heating lamps, radiant warmers, xenon lamps, and phototherapy lights may cause interference in SpO_2 measurements. It can be minimized by selecting correct probe, applying probe at appropriate location, and shielding the probe by coverings.
- *Electrical interference* from electrosurgical units can lead to false SpO_2 values along with incorrect pulse count.
- *Infrared interference* by neuronavigational equipment may alter SpO_2 values. To prevent it, the probe may be covered with aluminium foil.
- *Motion artifacts:* Although less common with newer generation pulse oximeters, motion artifacts such as occurring during transport of patients, Parkinson's disease, shivering, or during use of evoked potential monitors and nerve stimulators, may result in both false positive and false negative errors.

Various methods may be tried to improve the signal of pulse oximeters (**Box 3**).

> **BOX 3:** Methods to improve pulse oximeter signals.
>
> - Cover the hand, warm it by rubbing the skin
> - Careful sensor positioning on a different finger
> - Topical vasodilator application
> - Change the probe
> - Try a different probe site, e.g., ear
> - Change the machine
> - Use pulse oximeter with signal extraction technology

COMPLICATIONS

- *Pressure injuries:* Ranging from numbness to ischemic injury at the site of probe, usually due to the prolonged or tight application probe application, or compromised limb perfusion. Frequent site examination with changing of the probe site can help. Also, the probe should not be fixed circumferentially with tape.
- *Burns:* Although incidence is quite low, mild redness to third degree burn can result from incompatibility between the probe of one manufacturer and pulse oximeter of another manufacturer. Frequent site inspection and site rotation is recommended.
- *Skin irritation* can occur from adhesive on the probe.
- *Corneal abrasions* can result from inadvertent rubbing of eyes with probe on the finger.
- *Electric shock* is a very rare complication.

CONCLUSION

Being easy to use, noninvasive, accurate, and rapid, pulse oximetry forewarns the clinicians about early hypoxemia. Despite its limitations in patient-specific populations, it has revolutionized bedside oxygenation monitoring and represents a standard mandatory module for all critically ill patients.

SUGGESTED READING

1. Chan ED, Chan MM, Chan MM. Pulse oximetry: understanding its basic principles facilitates appreciation of its limitations. Respir Med. 2013;107:789-99.
2. Dorsch JA, Dorsch SE (Eds). A Practical Approach to Anesthesia Equipment. Philadelphia: Lippincott Williams & Wilkins; 2011.
3. Gropper MA, Eriksson LI, Fleisher LA, Wiener-Kronish JP, Cohen NH, Leslie K (Eds). Miller's Anesthesia, 9th edition. Netherlands: Elsevier; 2020.
4. Kamat V. Pulse oximetry. Indian J Anaesth. 2002;46:261-8.

Venous and Arterial Blood Gas Analysis

CHAPTER 15

Rajesh Pande, Maitree Pandey, Jitin Sharma

INTRODUCTION

As the name suggests, a sample drawn either from radial artery or a peripheral/central vein in a heparinized syringe is required for the analysis. Essentially, arterial blood gas (ABG) analysis provides information regarding acid–base status of the patient as well as about oxygenation and ventilation status in critical patients. It can also give us additional parameters like blood glucose, co-oximetry, electrolytes, and lactate vales depending on the capability of the ABG analyzer. The gold standard is an arterial sample drawn from a peripheral artery or an indwelling arterial catheter and gives comprehensive information, however there are situations when peripheral pulses are not palpable and there is no indwelling arterial catheter. In such situations, a peripheral or central venous sample is convenient, easier to obtain, and quite useful. It can provide information about pH, carbon dioxide (CO_2), bicarbonate (HCO_3^-) blood sugar, and electrolytes like an arterial sample. The differences between information obtained from venous and ABG analysis are listed in **Table 1**.

The popular physiological approach (Boston approach) uses the carbonic acid–bicarbonate buffer system to explain acid–base disorder. Although it is an oversimplistic approach, but easy to explain and understand. It identifies acids as hydrogen-ion donors and bases as hydrogen-ion acceptors. The carbonic acid–bicarbonate system is important in maintaining homeostatic control. A primary change in the partial pressure of carbon dioxide (PCO_2) causes a secondary compensatory response in the bicarbonate concentration and vice versa. Further changes in CO_2 or bicarbonate reflect additional changes in acid–base status. The four recognized primary acid–base disorders comprise two metabolic disorders (acidosis and alkalosis) and two respiratory disorders (acidosis and alkalosis). The common clinical conditions and associated acid–base disorders are listed in **Table 2**.

PaO_2 and $PaCO_2$: The inspired oxygen pressure (PiO_2) is 150 mm Hg $(760 - 47) \times 0.21$, where the atmospheric pressure is 760 mm Hg which contains water vapor with a pressure of 47 mm Hg. The alveolar pressure of oxygen (PAO_2) is about 100 mm Hg, and is measured using the alveolar gas equation: $PAO_2 = PiO_2 - PaCO_2/RQ$ ($150 - 40/0.8$). The alveolar–arterial

TABLE 1: Difference between arterial and venous blood gas.

	Arterial	Venous	A – V difference
pH	7.35–7.45	7.31–7.41	~0.04
PCO_2	35–45	41–51	~6
PO_2	80–100	30–40	~50
SaO_2 (%)	>95	75	>20
HCO_3^-	22–28	23–29	~1

TABLE 2: Common clinical conditions and associated acid–base disorders.

Clinical state	Acid–base disorder
Pulmonary embolus	Respiratory alkalosis
Hypotension	Metabolic acidosis
Vomiting	Metabolic alkalosis
Severe diarrhea	Metabolic acidosis
Cirrhosis	Respiratory alkalosis
Renal failure	Metabolic acidosis
Sepsis	Respiratory alkalosis, metabolic acidosis
Pregnancy	Respiratory alkalosis
Diuretic use	Metabolic alkalosis
COPD	Respiratory acidosis

(COPD: chronic obstructive pulmonary disease)

gradient (A-a gradient) is the difference between the partial pressure of oxygen in the alveoli and arterial system. The A-a gradient is calculated as: A-a Gradient = $PAO_2 - PaO_2$, where PAO_2 is the alveolar oxygen pressure and PaO_2 represents the arterial oxygen pressure. ABG assesses PaO_2 directly, and the difference is 10 mm Hg (100 - 90).

Normally in a perfect system, there should not be any A-a gradient. However, there is a difference in ventilation–perfusion (V/Q) of the apical and basal areas of the lung resulting in V/Q mismatch, which is considered physiological. This mismatch is, in part, responsible for the slight difference in oxygen tension between the alveoli and arterial blood. The expected A-a gradient can be calculated as: A-a gradient = (Age + 10)/4. The normal A-a gradient ranges from 5 to 25 mm Hg. However, the diffusion of oxygen from alveoli across the interstitium to the blood capillary also depends on the status of alveolar-interstitial-capillary complex, which is severely affected in conditions like pneumonia and acute respiratory distress syndrome (ARDS), where the PaO_2 is much lower than normal. PaO_2 <80 mm Hg represents hypoxemia and type I respiratory failure.

When a patient is breathing 100% oxygen and the measured PaO_2 is 55 mm Hg, $PaCO_2$ is 40 mm Hg, the PiO_2 and PAO_2 would be 760 mm Hg and 710 mm Hg, respectively and the A-a difference would be about 655 mm Hg, which indicates type I (hypoxemic) respiratory failure. A return in this value toward normalization indicates recovery from the disease. Normal partial pressure of oxygen (PO_2) ranges between 80 and 104 mm Hg on room air and PO_2 <80 mm Hg is hypoxemia. PO_2 decreases by 1 mm Hg below 80 mm Hg for every year of age above 60 years. The acceptable range in newborn is 40–70 mm Hg. A PaO_2/FiO_2 ratio >500 is considered as normal and between 300 and 500, there is some degree of oxygenation problem, but a value <300 represents hypoxemia. ARDS patients are classified into mild (200-300), moderate (100-200), and severe (≤100) ARDS based on P/F ratio, in addition to positive end-expiratory pressure (PEEP) of ≥5 cm H_2O and other criteria.

Similarly the $PaCO_2$ represents adequacy of ventilation and a rise in $PaCO_2$ >45 mm Hg is seen in acute exacerbation of chronic obstructive pulmonary disease (COPD), prolonged unresponsive exacerbation of asthma, permissive hypercapnia in ventilated ARDS, advanced ARDS, severe acute asthma, alveolar hypoventilation, central nervous system (CNS) depression, and thoracic cage restriction. The acute rise in CO_2 is associated with minimal compensation (for each 10 mm Hg rise in $PaCO_2$, the HCO_3 increases by 1 mEq), whereas in chronic respiratory acidosis for each 10 mm Hg rise in $PaCO_2$, the HCO_3 increases by 4. In acute respiratory acidosis, each 10 mm change in $PaCO_2$ also results in 0.08 decrease in pH ($\Delta pH = 0.008 \times \Delta PaCO_2$), whereas in chronic condition, each 10 mm change in $PaCO_2$ causes 0.03 decrease in pH ($\Delta pH = 0.003 \times \Delta PaCO_2$).

A fall in $PaCO_2$ below 35 mm Hg represents respiratory alkalosis, which could be due to high minute ventilation in ventilated patients. Similarly, in acute respiratory alkalosis, there is 2 mEq/L decrease in HCO_3 (below 24) for every 10 mm Hg decrease of PCO_2 below 40 (or $\Delta pH = 0.008 \times \Delta PaCO_2$) and expected pH = 7.4 + ΔpH. Similarly in chronic respiratory alkalosis, there is 5 mEq/L decrease in HCO_3 (below 24) for every 10 mm Hg decrease of PCO_2 below 40 (or the change in pH is represented as $\Delta pH = 0.003 \times (40 - PaCO_2)$ and expected pH = 7.4 + ΔpH. The causes of respiratory alkalosis are listed in **Box 1**. The compensatory secondary responses in respiratory disorders generally take 2–5 days.

Arterial blood gas also provides important information about the metabolic status of the patient. Human body continuously produces acids (H^+ ion donors). The normal diet generates volatile acids (CO_2) from carbohydrate and nonvolatile acids (H^+) from protein metabolism. Our lungs and kidneys are responsible for maintaining acid–base homeostasis by excreting these acids. The alveolar ventilation allows for excretion of CO_2. Human kidney reclaims all the filtered HCO_3^-. Any urinary loss of bicarbonate would lead to net gain of H^+. The kidneys also excrete the daily protein load generated from protein intake and less than half of acid load is excreted as titrable acids (phosphoric and sulfuric acids) and remaining is excreted as NH_4^+. This process increases markedly in metabolic acidosis. Buffers and respiration are temporary mechanisms, whereas kidneys can make permanent adjustments. The relationship between H^+ ion and pH and bicarbonate conservation by kidneys are explained in **Figures 1 and 2**, respectively. Consistency of

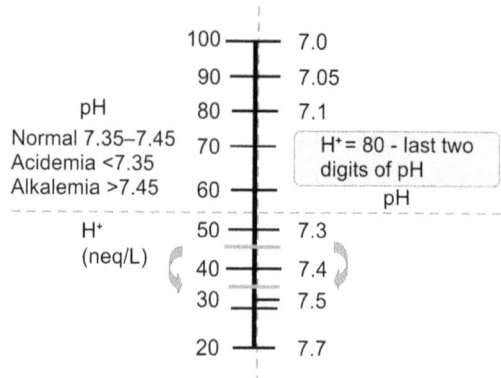

Fig. 1: Relationship between H^+ ion and pH.

the ABG result can be verified by calculating H^+ using the Henderson–Hasselbalch equation. $H^+ = 24 \times (PaCO_2 \div HCO_3^-)$. If HCO_3^- is 12 and $PaCO_2$ is 35, then the H^+ concentration = $24 \times (35 \div 12) = 70$, and the increase in H^+ = 70 − 40 = 30 **(Fig. 1)**. For every 1 nEq/L change in H^+ from 40, there is a 0.01 change from 7.4 in the opposite direction. Therefore $\Delta pH = 30 \times 0.01 = 0.3$ and the change in pH is 7.4 − 0.3 = 7.1. If it matches with the pH of ABG sample, then data is internally consistent.

Henderson–Hasselbalch equation forms the basis for using bicarbonate–carbonic acid buffer system to diagnose acid–base disorders.

$$pH = 6.1 + \log HCO_3^-/(PaCO_2 \times 0.03)$$
$$H^+ = 24 \times PaCO_2/HCO_3^-$$

Bicarbonate–carbonic acid buffer system is the principal extracellular buffer and the most important.

$$(H_2O + CO_2 \leftrightarrow H_2CO_3 \leftrightarrow H^+ + HCO_3^-)$$

Adding acid load to the body consumes HCO_3^-. The CO_2 is maintained within a narrow range via respiratory drive and the HCO_3^- is regenerated by the kidneys. Primary changes in $PaCO_2$ lead to respiratory acidosis or alkalosis, whereas the primary changes in HCO_3^- lead to metabolic acidosis or alkalosis. $PaCO_2$ and HCO_3^- move in the same direction

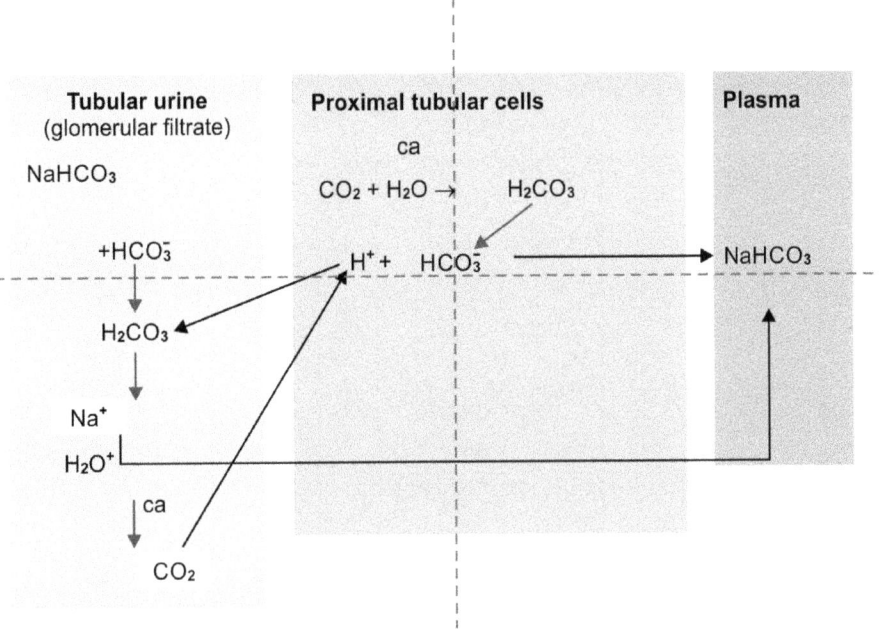

Fig. 2: Bicarbonate conservation by kidneys.

in simple disorders. In metabolic acidosis bicarbonate–carbonic acid is the first buffer to come in action and after all the HCO_3 is reclaimed by kidneys and still the H load is high, H^+ secreted into renal tubules can combine with phosphate ions (HPO_4^-) to form H_2PO_4 which is eliminated in urine. NH_3/NH_4 pair becomes the most important buffer after bicarbonate–carbonic acid and phosphate buffers have been utilized. Ammonia comes from deamination of glutamine in proximal tubular cells and combines with H^+ to form ammonium (NH_4^+), which is removed in urine.

Metabolic acidosis results in decrease in pH below 7.35 and increase in H^+ ions >40 mEq **(Table 1)**.

Compensation for metabolic acidosis occurs by wash out of CO_2 (increase in ventilation) and can be calculated by Winter's formula (predicted $PaCO_2 = 1.5 \times [HCO_3^-] + 8 \pm 2$). The compensatory mechanisms take 12–24 hours. One should also look for presence of anion gap (AG) which is the difference between measured cations and anions **(Fig. 3)**. It helps us in differentiating whether metabolic acidosis is due to H^+ ions accumulation or loss of HCO_3^- ions.

$$AG = Na^+ - (Cl^- + HCO_3^-)$$

It is usually <12; if >12, it is labeled as AG acidosis. The normal range is 10 ± 4 mEq/L. However, it is affected by the albumin level and in hypoalbuminemia, actual AG is higher than measured and albumin correction needs to be applied (add 1 to the AG for every gram change in albumin from normal).

Albumin correction: Adjusted AG = 10 + 2.5 (normal serum albumin − measured albumin)

For example, if AG is 10 and serum albumin is 2. The adjusted AG would be 12.5 {10 + (4.5 − 2)}.

The causes of AG and non-AG metabolic acidosis are listed in **Boxes 2 and 3**, respectively.

Whenever there is metabolic acidosis, we should check whether there is a wide

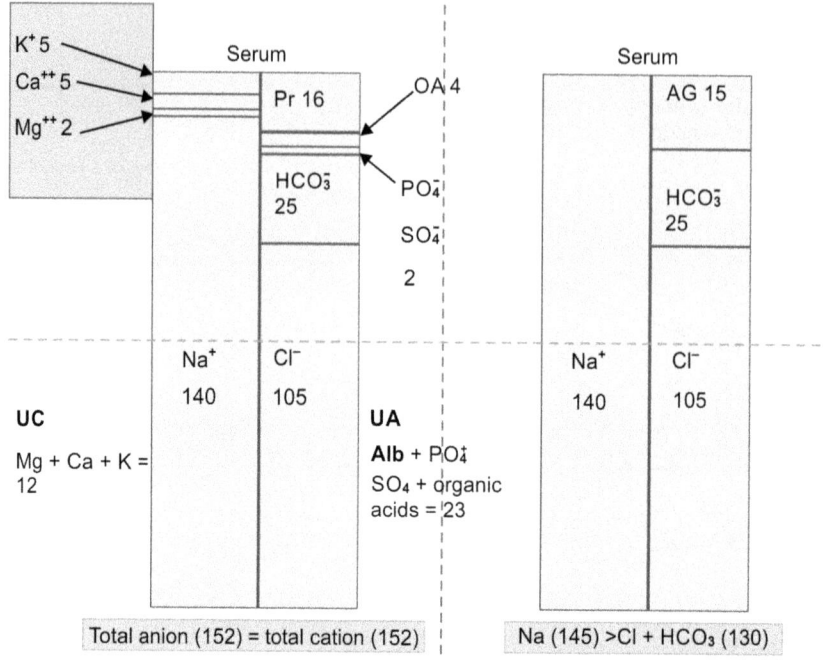

Fig. 3: Concept of anion gap.

AG. The causes of high AG metabolic acidosis include: organic source—lactic acidosis, ketoacidosis, renal failure, increased production of endogenous nonvolatile acids; ingestion of toxins—methanol, ethylene glycol, salicylate, and exogenous nonvolatile acids.

The causes of high AG metabolic acidosis include {pneumonic MUDPILES [methanol, uremia, diabetic ketoacidosis (DKA) (or alcoholic ketoacidosis), paraldehyde, iron (or isoniazid), lactic acidosis, ethylene glycol, and salicylates]} are listed in **Box 1**.

In high AG metabolic acidosis, the next step is to look at ΔAG and ΔHCO$_3$ gap, and at the gap-gap ratio: ΔAG/ΔHCO$_3$. It assesses the elevation of the AG relative to the decrease in HCO$_3^-$. Normal value is 1–1.6. If it is <1, it indicates that HCO$_3^-$ has decreased out of proportion to the elevation of AG and concomitant non-AG metabolic acidosis is present. If it is >1.6, the AG has increased out of proportion to the rise in HCO$_3^-$ and concomitant metabolic alkalosis is present.

Whenever there is a normal AG metabolic acidosis, one should look at relationship between chloride and sodium. Normal Cl$^-$ (105): Na$^+$ (140) ratio = 1:1.4 and if >1:1.14,

BOX 1: Causes of respiratory alkalosis.

- Hypoxemia
- Mechanical ventilation
- Central causes
- Fever
- Anxiety
- Hormones—catecholamine, progesterone
- Drugs—salicylates, analeptics
- Sepsis
- Hyperthyroidism
- Pregnancy
- Cirrhosis
- Pulmonary edema
- Pulmonary embolism
- Pneumonia

> **BOX 2:** Causes of high anion gap metabolic acidosis.
>
> M = Methanol
> U = Uremia
> D = Diabetic ketoacidosis
> P = Paraldehyde
> I = Infection
> L = Lactic acid
> E = Ethylene glycol
> R = Rhabdomyolysis, renal failure
> S = Salicylate

> **BOX 3:** Causes of normal anion gap metabolic acidosis.
>
> H = Hyperalimentation
> A = Acetazolamide
> R = Renal tubular acidosis
> D = Diarrhea, enterocutaneous fistulas
> U = Uremia (acute)
> P = Post ventilation hypocapnia
> S = Saline infusion

it is called hyperchloremic metabolic acidosis. Normally a loss of HCO_3^- is counterbalanced by a gain in chloride and the AG remains normal.

Causes of hyperchloremic metabolic acidosis include: diarrhea [increased gastrointestinal (GI) losses of HCO_3^-], increased renal loss of HCO_3^- [Type II renal tubular acidosis (RTA)], failure to excrete H^+ (Type I RTA), dilutional (large volume infusion of saline, amino acids, NH_4Cl infusion), and other less common causes like short bowel syndrome, pancreatic fistula, fistula between ureter and GI tract, and recovery from DKA.

The acidemia algorithm is explained in **Flowchart 1**.

When the pH is increased >7.4, indicating reduction in H^+ and a rise in HCO_3 it is called metabolic alkalosis. Here the compensation is by a rise in $PaCO_2$.

The expected $PaCO_2 = 0.7 [HCO_3] + 20 (\pm 5)$. The compensation takes 24–36 hours. Metabolic alkalosis could be the result of chloride responsive (urinary chloride <15 mEq/L) or nonresponsive (urine chloride >25 mEq/L) causes. For chloride responsive metabolic alkalosis, saline infusion can be used for correction. Chloride deficit (mEq) is calculated as $0.3 \times$ Wt. (kg) $\times (100 - $ plasma $Cl^-)$. The volume of isotonic saline (L) is chloride deficit/154. For chloride unresponsive metabolic alkalosis, the hypokalemia should be corrected, and mineralocorticoid and glucocorticoid excess should be controlled. Algorithm for alkalemia and chloride responsiveness are explained in **Flowchart 2** and **Table 3**.

Some precautions are required during the conduct and processing of an arterial ABG sample. Blood should be collected and transported without exposure to air (i.e., collected anaerobically), otherwise PaO_2 will increase. There should not be any air as it can also cause a slight increase in pH and decrease in pCO_2. Once the sample is drawn, it should be mixed thoroughly by inverting the syringe several times and rolling it between the palms of the hands. One should be careful as excess heparin can cause red blood cell (RBC) hemolysis, reducing pH, PCO_2 and PO_2.

Boston formulae are based on the bicarbonate-carbonic acid system and any change in respiratory acid also causes a change in the baseline used for assessment of metabolic disorder affecting the analysis of complex acid–base disorders. The Copenhagen approach is based on several $PaCO_2$ independent indices like base excess (BE), standard bicarbonate, and buffer base.

Base excess is defined as the amount of acid (H^+) or base (HCO_3^-) that must be added to 1 L of whole blood to return blood pH to 7.40 and $PaCO_2$ to 40 mm Hg at full O_2 saturation and 37°C. (Deviation of patient's HCO_3^- from 24 mmol/L after pH is corrected to 7.4). It is usually derived from a monogram. A negative value indicates metabolic acidosis and a

Flowchart 1: Workup of academia.

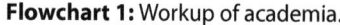

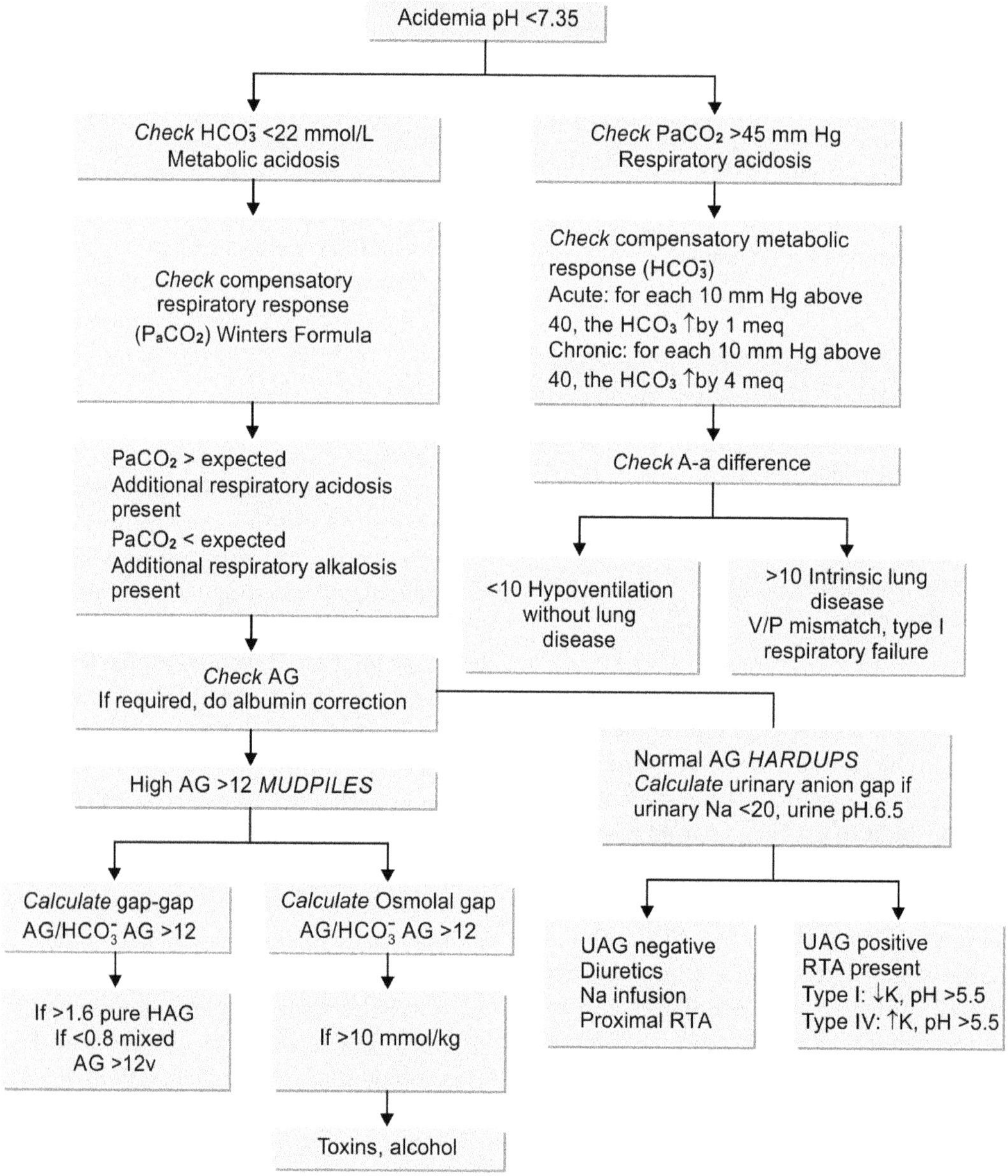

```
                        Acidemia pH <7.35
                              │
              ┌───────────────┴───────────────┐
              ▼                               ▼
   Check HCO₃ <22 mmol/L              Check PaCO₂ >45 mm Hg
   Metabolic acidosis                  Respiratory acidosis
              │                               │
              ▼                               ▼
   Check compensatory           Check compensatory metabolic
   respiratory response         response (HCO₃)
   (PaCO₂) Winters Formula      Acute: for each 10 mm Hg above
                                40, the HCO₃ ↑ by 1 meq
                                Chronic: for each 10 mm Hg above
                                40, the HCO₃ ↑ by 4 meq
              │                               │
              ▼                               ▼
   PaCO₂ > expected             Check A-a difference
   Additional respiratory acidosis
   present
   PaCO₂ < expected
   Additional respiratory alkalosis
   present                          ┌──────────┴──────────┐
              │                     ▼                     ▼
              ▼              <10 Hypoventilation    >10 Intrinsic lung
        Check AG             without lung           disease
  If required, do albumin correction  disease       V/P mismatch, type I
              │                                     respiratory failure
              │                     Normal AG HARDUPS
              │                     Calculate urinary anion gap if
              ▼                     urinary Na <20, urine pH.6.5
   High AG >12 MUDPILES
```

Calculate gap-gap	Calculate Osmolal gap	UAG negative	UAG positive
AG/HCO₃ AG >12	AG/HCO₃ AG >12	Diuretics	RTA present
		Na infusion	Type I: ↓K, pH >5.5
If >1.6 pure HAG	If >10 mmol/kg	Proximal RTA	Type IV: ↑K, pH >5.5
If <0.8 mixed			
AG >12v	Toxins, alcohol		

(AG: anion gap; HAG: high anion gap; HARDUPS: hyperalimentation, acetazolamide, renal tubular acidosis, diarrhea, enterocutaneous fistulas, uremia (acute), post ventilation hypocapnia, saline infusion; MUDPILES: methanol, uremia, diabetic ketoacidosis (DKA) (or alcoholic ketoacidosis), paraldehyde, iron (or isoniazid), lactic acidosis, ethylene glycol, and salicylates; RTA: renal tubular acidosis; UAG: urine anion gap)

Notes: Albumin correction for AG = for every 1 g/dL albumin decrease, increase calculated AG by 2.5 mmol/L
Urinary anion gap = $Na^+ + K^+ - Cl^-$
Calculated osmolality = $(2 \times [Na^+]) + [\text{glucose in mg/dL}]/18 + (\text{BUN in mg/dL})/2.8$
Osmolal gap = Measured − Calculated osmolality

CHAPTER 15: Venous and Arterial Blood Gas Analysis

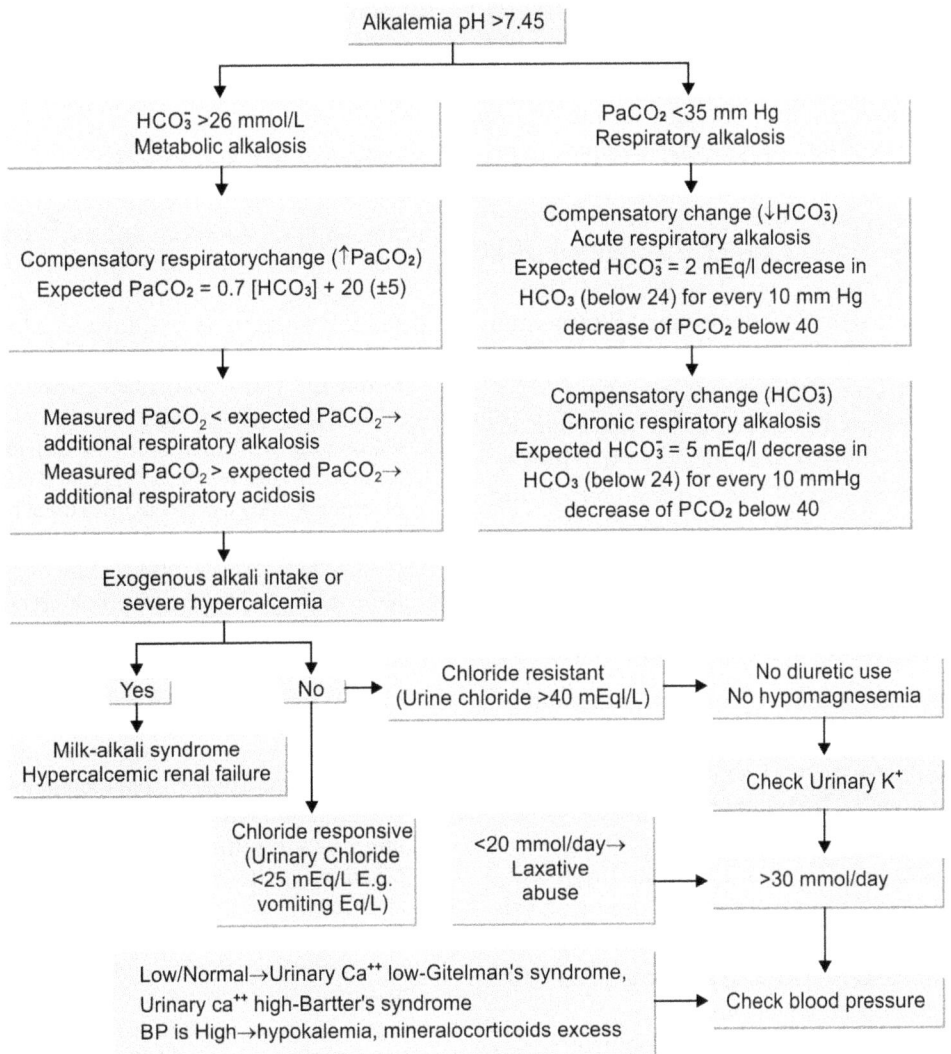

Flowchart 2: Algorithm for management of alkalemia.

Chloride responsive	Chloride unresponsive
Due to vomiting/nasogratsic tube aspiration	Potassium depletion
Diuretics (long-term use)	Diuretics (recent use)
Volume depletion	Mineralocorticoid excess
Chloride losing diarrhea	Primary hyperaldosteronism
Posthypercapnia	Cushing's disease
	Ectopic ACTH

TABLE 3: Chloride responsive and unresponsive metabolic alkalosis.

(ACTH: adrenocorticotropic hormone; NG: nasogastric)

positive value indicates metabolic alkalosis. BE calculation takes hemoglobin (Hb) of 5 g/dL represents the Hb of the whole extracellular fluid (ECF) if the Hb is distributed throughout the ECF rather than just being confined to the intravascular compartment. This removes the bias that buffering of blood is the same as the buffering by the whole ECF.

Buffer base is a measure of the concentration of *all* the buffers present in either plasma or blood. Blood buffer base is practically the sum of bicarbonate, albumin, and Hb, which is about 48 mmol/L in normal subjects.

Standard BE or base deficit (BD): It is an ideal metabolic index independent of $PaCO_2$.

Base excess or BD is corrected for Hb and size of interstitial fluid compartment. It can be calculated by dividing BE by 3 or calculating BE using Hb of 5 g/dL.

$$SBE = 0.93 \times ([HCO_3^-] + 14.48 \times [pH - 7.4] - 24.4$$

Reference range = –3 to +3 mEq/L. Standard bicarbonate is the bicarbonate concentration of a sample when the pCO_2 has been adjusted (or "standardized") to 40 mm Hg at a temperature of 37°C. This would remove the influence of changes in pCO_2 by seeing what the $[HCO_3]$ would be if the respiratory component was made the same for all measurements. Standard HCO_3^- decreases in metabolic acidosis and increases in metabolic alkalosis.

It is important to understand that a stepwise approach helps in understanding the acid–base disorders. The ABG report should always be clinically correlated with the patient condition. Another method is the strong ion or Stewart approach which is outside the scope of this chapter and is not discussed.

SUGGESTED READING

1. Berend K, de Vries APJ, Gans ROB. Physiological approach to assessment of acid–base disturbances. N Engl J Med. 2014; 371:1434-45.
2. Brito V, Spiegler P, Upadhyay S. Understanding the limitations of your arterial blood gas (ABG) analysis. Chest. 2012; 142(4_MeetingAbstracts):313A.
3. DellaVolpe JD, Chakraborti C, Cerreta K, Romero CJ, Firestein CE, Myers L, et al. Effects of implementing a protocol for arterial blood gas use on ordering practices and diagnostic yield. Healthc (Amst). 2014;2(2):130-5.
4. Melanson SEF, Szymanski T, Rogers SO, Jarolim P, Frendl G, Rawn JD, et al. Utilization of arterial blood gas measurements in a large tertiary care hospital. Am J Clin Pathol. 2007;127(4):604-9.
5. Merlani P, Garnerin P, Diby M, Ferring M, Ricou B. Quality improvement report linking guideline to regular feedback to increase appropriate requests for clinical tests: blood gas analysis in intensive care. BMJ. 2001;323:620-4.
6. Pande RK. Arterial blood gas: bowling wide and poor wicketkeeping. Indian J Crit Care Med. 2021;25(2):119-20.
7. Salam A, Smina M, Gada P, Tilluckdharry L, Upadya A, Amoateng-Adjepong Y, et al. The effect of arterial blood gas values on extubation decisions. Respir Care. 2003;48(11):1033-7.

SECTION 3: Oxygen Delivery Systems for the Individual Patients

- **Oxygen-Delivery Devices**
  Tapas Kumar Sahoo, Santanu Bagchi, Rajesh Chandra

- **Humidification**
  Vikram Damaraju, Inderpaul Sehgal

- **High-Flow Nasal Cannula**
  Harjit Dumra, Mansi Dandnaik

- **Hyperbaric Oxygen Therapy**
  Gunjan Chanchalani, Sunil Amin, Kanwalpreet Sodhi

- **Oxygen Toxicity**
  Shrikant Sahasrabudhe, Beena Daniel

Oxygen-Delivery Devices

CHAPTER

Tapas Kumar Sahoo, Santanu Bagchi, Rajesh Chandra

INTRODUCTION

The first thing that we need to remember about oxygen therapy is that it is no different from a drug therapy and therefore, oxygen therapy has its indications, contraindications, dosing, specific physiochemical effects, adverse effects, etc. There comes the responsibility of the caregivers regarding the optimization of this therapy, which more than often is being used as a life saver. Tissue oxygenation is dependent on both oxygen delivery to the tissues and oxygen utilization by the tissues. Our discussion would be limited to the first component, i.e., oxygen delivery. Now, if we go back to physiology, oxygen delivery to the tissues is an integrated function involving cardiopulmonary and hematological systems. The beginning starts with fortifying the inhaled air with oxygen to increase its concentration and that is the essence of oxygen therapy—delivering the patient an oxygen concentration which is greater than that of ambient air.

OXYGEN-DELIVERY DEVICES

There are different types of oxygen-delivery devices with unique features. The choice of the delivery system may be based on multiple factors such as degree of hypoxemia, requirement for precision of delivery, and patient comfort. These devices can be classified in several manners. One of the ways in which these devices can be broadly classified is either variable-performance devices (low-flow devices) or fixed-performance devices (high-flow devices) **(Flowchart 1)**.

The low-flow devices cannot deliver a constant fraction of inspired oxygen (FiO_2) as it varies with a tidal volume and consequently gets diluted with the ambient air. On the

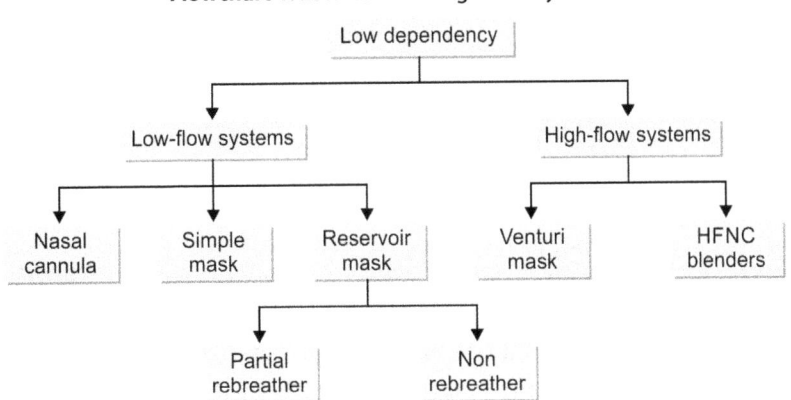

Flowchart 1: Low-flow and high-flow systems.

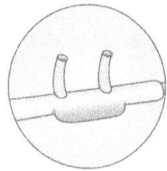 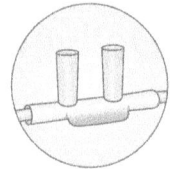 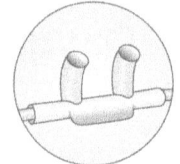 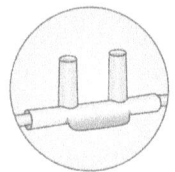 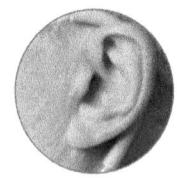

Curved prongs: Improved anatomical fit

Flared prongs: Slows down the flow of oxygen

Curved/flared prongs: Combines the of curved and flared designs

Straight prongs

Curved prongs with ear guards: Improved anatomical fit and patient comfort

Fig. 1: Different prong shapes and sizes.

other hand, high-flow devices can maintain a constant FiO_2 and deliver oxygen at a higher flow which is usually four times of the actual minute volume of the individual. Therefore, patients with higher hypoxic drive—or, in other words, in profound type one respiratory failure—would benefit from fixed-performance devices delivering higher and controlled increments in FiO_2.

Common low-flow devices include nasal cannula, nasal catheters, transtracheal catheter, face mask, partial rebreathing mask, nonrebreathing mask, tracheostomy mask, etc.

Nasal Cannula

Nasal cannula consists of two soft prongs attached to the oxygen supply tubing. A flow rate of 1–6 L/min delivers a fraction of inspired oxygen (FiO_2) of 0.24–0.40. The calculation can be done with the following formula:

$$FiO_2 = 20\% + (4 \times \text{oxygen liter flow})$$

Nasopharynx acts as a reservoir. If the flow is >6 L/min, there happens to be no increase in FiO_2. If the patient breathes through their mouth, air flow produces a Venturi effect in the posterior pharynx, entraining oxygen from the nose. Nasal cannula is available in different sizes and different prong shapes **(Fig. 1)**.

The problem with nasal cannula use lies in the risk of nasal mucosal drying and epistaxis

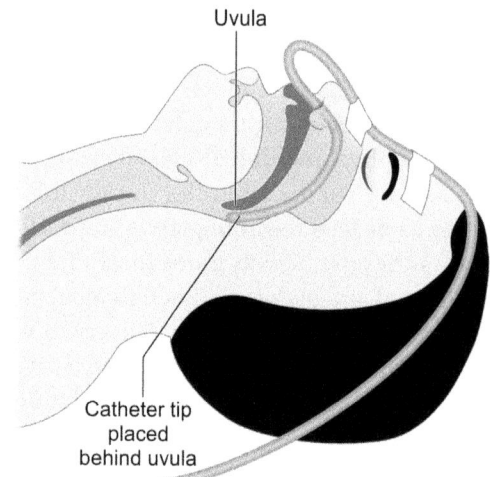

Fig. 2: Nasal catheter.

on prolonged use. Moreover, its primary limitation lies in its inability to provide higher oxygenation and also higher effective flow, if a patient needs the same. The user-friendly interface with independence to the patient regarding talking, eating, or even mobilizing while being on nasal cannula for mild oxygen therapy, its light weight and low cost all can be counted as advantages of nasal cannula.

Nasal Catheter

Nasal catheter is a single-lumen catheter, which is lodged into the anterior nares by a foam collar, inserted just above the uvula **(Fig. 2)**. In this device also, the oxygen flow would be limited, usually 2–3 L/min. Additional significant disadvantages include the risk of gastric distention by air in the event of deep insertion and contraindication of its use in a situation of suspected mucosal tear. This catheter must be repositioned every 8 hours to prevent its breakdown. In general, it has no advantages over nasal cannula, with those above-mentioned drawbacks.

Simple Face Mask

A face mask can provide a higher oxygen supply compared to nasal cannula/catheters **(Fig. 3)**. This happens because it can provide an additional reservoir of 100–200 mL. It gets fitted over the nose and the mouth of the patient; the oxygen reaches the mask through an attached pipe and carbon dioxide (CO_2) gets exhaled via the side ports. Therefore, any mask's efficiency depends on how well it fits over and for the same reason, its use is limited in the events of facial injury and burns. It can be set to deliver 5–10 L/min oxygen (FiO_2 0.35–0.55). A minimum of 5 L/min flow is needed to prevent the rebreathing of CO_2.

The patient may feel claustrophobic while being on mask, and eating and drinking would also be difficult. These masks are kept transparent in order to identify any vomitus or regurgitation or bleeding early. Any inadvertent eye injury arising from the mask position needs to be taken care of.

Partial Rebreather Face Mask

In this type of face mask, a reservoir bag is attached with a capacity of 1 L (adult) and as the name suggests, it allows partial rebreathing of exhaled CO_2 gas **(Fig. 4)**. Oxygen flows

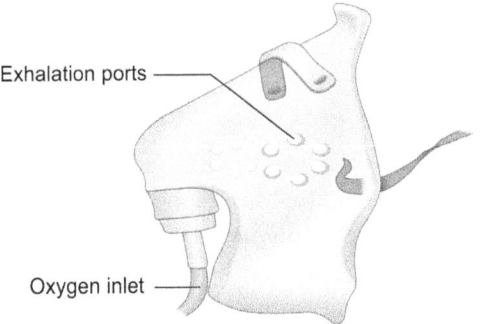

Fig. 3: Simple face mask.

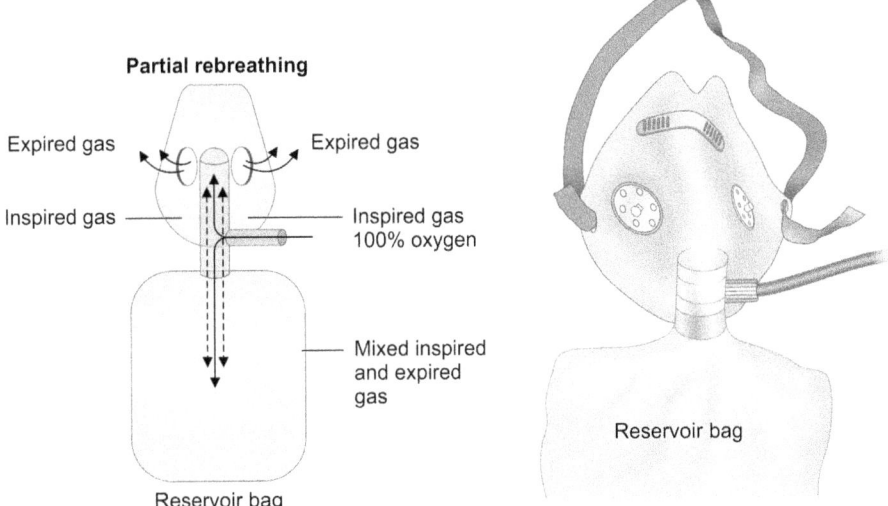

Fig. 4: Partial rebreather face mask.

directly into the reservoir bag and the exhaled gas from the initial part of expiration, which effectively comes from anatomic dead space, gets collected into the reservoir bag. The fresh gas flow (i.e., oxygen) thus needs to be kept on the higher side in order to keep the reservoir bag always inflated so that adequate oxygen gets delivered along with adequate evacuation of CO_2. This mask is particularly more useful in situations where oxygen supply is low, resulting in oxygen conservation. It provides an FiO_2 of 0.6–0.8 and requires a flow of minimum 8 L/min in order to keep the reservoir bag at least half-inflated. This mask also interferes with eating and drinking. Moreover, higher than the stipulated oxygen flow does not effectively increase the FiO_2.

Nonrebreather Mask

Additional factor in this type of face mask is the presence of a one-way valve between the mask interface and the reservoir bag **(Fig. 5)**. This one-way valve ensures unidirectional gaseous flow and thus exhaled gases get prevented from entering the reservoir bag, which in turn can act as a more pure source of oxygen, minimizing the rebreathing issue. This mask has got two side ports with a flutter valve, which prevents room air entrainment. Therefore, this mask can provide a significantly higher FiO_2 compared to other face masks in the range up to 0.95 with a flow of 10–15 L. In this mask, the minimum flow should be 10 L/min in order to keep the reservoir bag at least half-inflated. The advantage of this mask lies in its ability to deliver higher oxygen while the drawbacks are possibility of CO_2 retention in case of valve malfunction and the patient's discomfort due to prolonged use with a tight seal.

Transtracheal Oxygen Catheter

Transtracheal oxygen catheters, as the name suggests, are placed inside the trachea using the Seldinger technique via the percutaneous route **(Fig. 6)**. These can be useful in alleviating hypoxemia and respiratory distress. However,

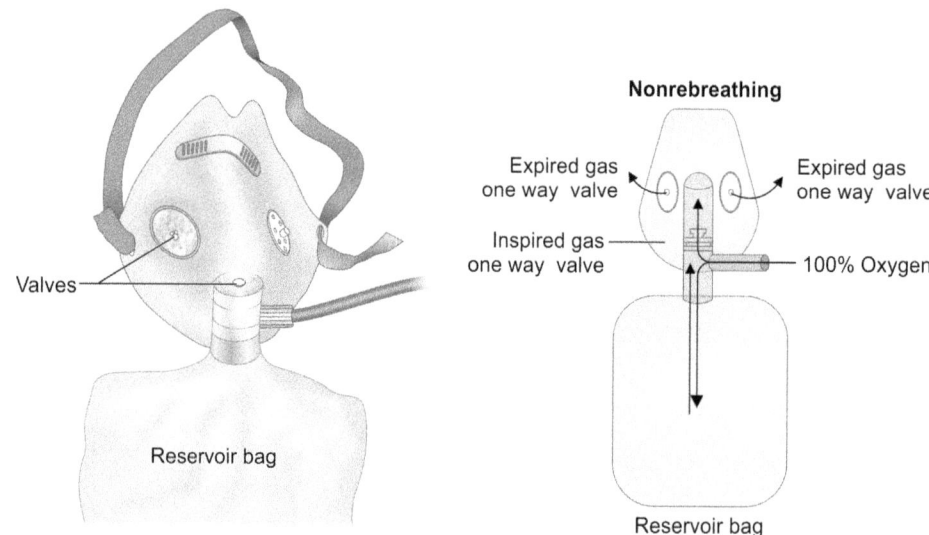

Fig. 5: Nonrebreathing mask.

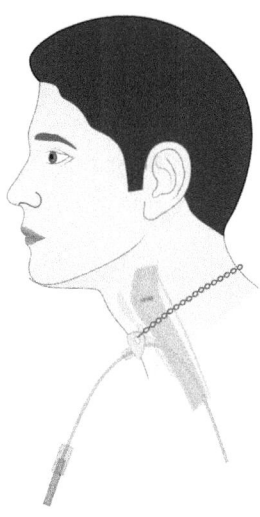

Fig. 6: Transtracheal oxygen catheter.

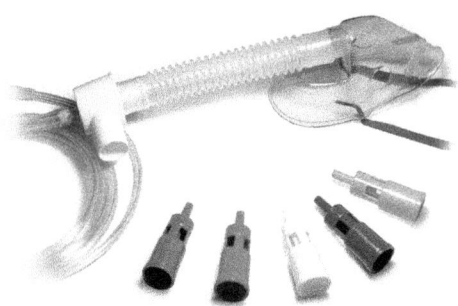

Fig. 7: Venturi mask.

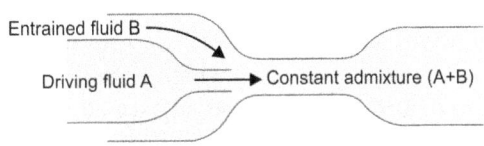

Fig. 8: Venturi principle.

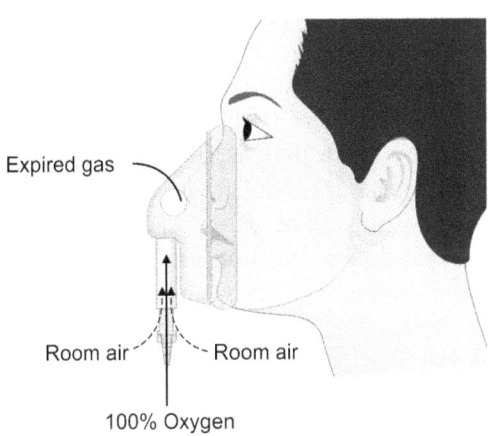

Fig. 9: Venturi mask functionality.

because of the sheer invasiveness and the patient's discomfort, this technique has not gained popularity. Moreover, there has been a lack of training and expertise regarding the usage of these catheters. The oxygen flow is usually between 0.5 and 4.0 L/min. The advantage of these catheters lies in avoiding the anatomical dead space of the upper airway and direct delivery of oxygen into the trachea. Therefore, the oxygen delivery percentage remains lower than other noninvasive measures.

Venturi Mask

Venturi mask belongs to the class of fixed-performance oxygen-delivery devices **(Fig. 7)**. It usually delivers a fixed concentration of oxygen, and the size of the constriction inside the Venturi device acts as the determining factor of final oxygen concentration for a given flow. The name of the mask originates from its functional mechanism which, in turn, is based on the Venturi modification of Bernoulli's principle **(Fig. 8)**. Structurally, the proximal end of the mask comprises a Venturi device which is color-coded and each device has its own designated oxygen flow rate, written on the device itself **(Fig. 9)**. The highest FiO_2 achievement is with a green color-coded device, providing an FiO_2 of 60%. Subsequently, in decreasing order, there are red, yellow, orange, white, and

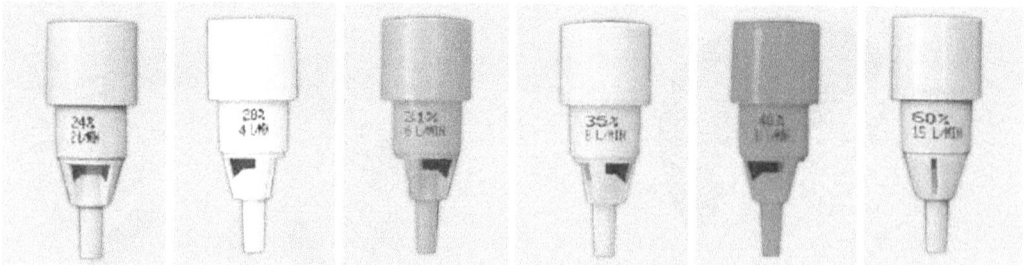

Fig. 10: Color-coded Venturi devices.

blue color-coded devices, which respectively deliver 40, 35, 31, 28, and 24% FiO_2 **(Fig. 10)**. However, there is a variable FiO_2 format of the Venturi mask also, which is not color-coded, and here a graded adjustment of air entrainment port can be done, which in turn would allow variable delivered FiO_2.

The advantage of a Venturi mask lies in the fact that it allows precise oxygen delivery, not a high FiO_2 delivery in general. Therefore, it is particularly useful in chronic inflammatory lung disease (COPD) patients where precise oxygen delivery is important. The fundamental mechanism of action depends on the principle of air entrainment. As the forward flow of inspired gas increases, the lateral pressure adjacent and perpendicular to the vector of flow decreases, resulting in the entrainment of gas. The smaller the orifice is, the greater the pressure drop where negative pressure is generated and more ambient air entrained and the lower the FiO_2. Due to the high fresh gas flow rate, the exhaled gases are rapidly flushed from the mask via its holes and therefore there is no rebreathing and no increase in the dead space. The oxygen flow exceeds the patient's peak expiratory flow. Therefore, it is unlikely for the patient to breathe in air from the room. This mask is also associated with eating and drinking interference and a sense of claustrophobia by some patients.

High-Flow Nasal Cannula

High-flow nasal cannula (HFNC) is an advancement in oxygen therapy modality where the patient's comfort meets classically with effective higher oxygen supplementation **(Fig. 11)**. The oxygen reaches the nasal cannula from the air–oxygen blender with the help of a flow generator. The advantage of the flow generator is that it can generate a much higher than usual flow, up to 60 L/min, which is particularly helpful in patients with a higher work of breathing in order to meet their demand. On the other hand, the blender can deliver up to 100% FiO_2 depending on the requirement. The device assembly also consists of a humidifier, which saturates the inflowing gas mix and thus provides much-needed humidification and ambient warmth (31–37°C) beneficial for the upper airway mucosa **(Fig. 12)**.

The physiologic mechanisms, believed to be responsible for the efficacy of HFNC, are multifaceted, including physiological dead space washout of waste gases, mild variable positive end-expiratory pressure effect (about 5 cm of H_2O), reduction in the respiratory rate, increase in the tidal volume, and reduction in the airflow resistance.

The HFNC, in addition to its ability of delivering a higher flow and FiO_2, due to being heated and humidified, provides patient

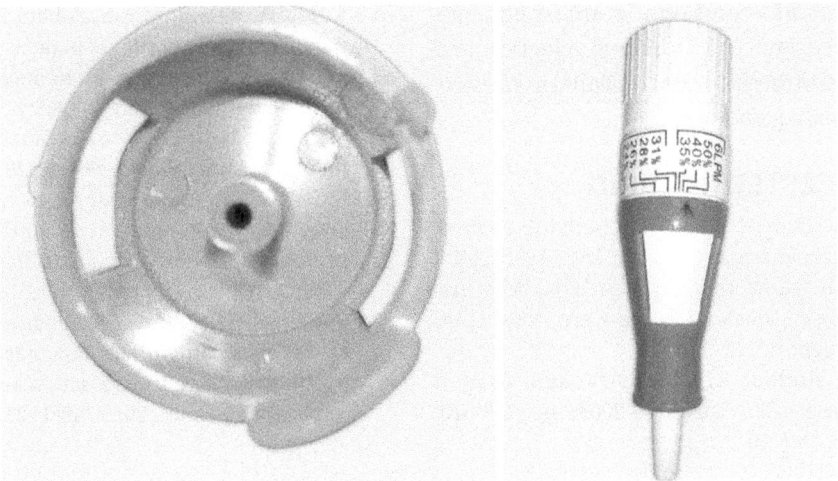

Fig. 11: High-flow nasal cannula.

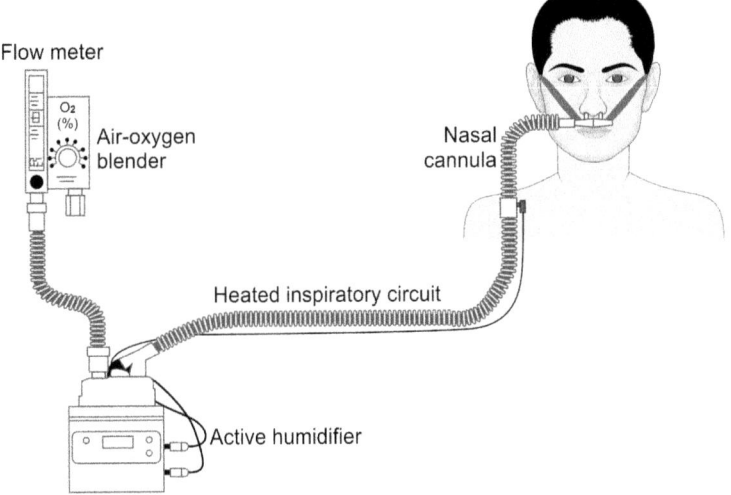

Fig. 12: High-flow nasal cannula.

comfort and independence of carrying out normal activities such as eating and drinking on the bed without feeling claustrophobic. The high flow and humidification greatly improve both the functional residual capacity and the mucociliary clearance of secretions and thus reduce the work of breathing. Overall, this device has been a valuable addition in the armamentarium for the management of hypoxic patients with respiratory distress.

CONCLUSION

Oxygen therapy is an essential and often lifesaving modality of therapy for a patient irrespective of their underlying condition and location of care. There have been different devices for this purpose and each of them has their unique characteristics, advantages, and limitations. The choice of oxygen therapy device can depend on multiple factors such as degree of hypoxemia, underlying pathophysiology of the patient's condition, at times patient's preference, etc. The judicious selection and utilization of these devices is pivotal in effective patient management, overall.

SUGGESTED READING

1. Bitterman H. Bench-to-bedside review: oxygen as a drug. Crit Care. 2009;13(1):205.
2. Chan YK, Ng KP, Sim DSM (Eds). Pharmacological Basis of Acute Care. New York: Springer; 2015.
3. Christopher KL. Transtracheal oxygen catheters. Clin Chest Med. 2003;24(3):489-510.
4. Korupolu R, Gifford J, Needham DM. Early mobilization of critically ill patients: reducing neuromuscular complications after intensive care. Contemp Crit Care. 2009;6:1-12.
5. Nishimura M. High-flow nasal cannula oxygen therapy in adults. J Intensive Care 2015;3(1):15.
6. Scacci R. Air entrainment masks: jet mixing is how they work; the Venturi and Bernoulli principles are how they don't. Respir Care. 1979;24:928-31.
7. Spoletini G, Alotaibi M, Blasi F, Hill NS. Heated humidified high-flow nasal oxygen in adults: mechanisms of action and clinical implications. Chest. 2015;148(1):253-61.

Humidification

CHAPTER 17

Vikram Damaraju, Inderpaul Sehgal

INTRODUCTION

Oxygen therapy is required for patients with hypoxemia (in and out of the hospital setting); however, as with other drugs, it is associated with adverse effects if not delivered appropriately. The provision of humidified oxygen improves patient comfort. There are different types of humidification systems available. However, patient and equipment-related factors (including risk and benefit) must be considered before selecting the appropriate humidification system.

PHYSIOLOGY

The upper respiratory tract is lined by pseudostratified ciliated columnar epithelium, mucus-secreting goblet cells, and capillaries. The function of cilia (bathed in mucus) is to effectively filter out dust particles, which are later expelled by coughing or sneezing. Additionally, the mucus secreted by goblet cells moistens the inspired air. The inspired air at room temperature is warmed by the blood capillaries lining the upper respiratory tract. Thus, inspired air reaching the alveoli is heated, humidified, and filtered. During expiration, the lining epithelium retains some heat and moisture for proper functioning.

HUMIDITY

The composition of the mucus and the ciliary movement is dependent on the ambient temperature and humidity. Humidity is the amount of water held by a gas. It can be described either as absolute or relative. Absolute humidity (AH) is the amount of water the gas holds (mg/L). The relative humidity (RH) is the ratio of water the gas holds compared to its total water holding capacity at a given temperature (measured as %). When the inspired air reaches the alveoli, it is heated to a body temperature of 37°C, with a RH of 100% and AH of approximately 44 mg/L.

HUMIDIFICATION OF OXYGEN THERAPY

The stored and supplied oxygen used for providing oxygen therapy is cold and dry. The cold and dry oxygen causes respiratory tract mucosa to dry out and hampers the airway cilia from filtering out dust particles. The dust particles impact the airway mucosa and thicken the secretions causing airway obstruction, increased airway resistance, and work of breathing. The cold and dry oxygen also causes nasal and oral dryness, epistaxis, burning sensation, speaking difficulty, and thirst. At high-flow rates, nonhumidified oxygen causes metaplasia and keratinization of the nasal mucosa. Humidification is required during invasive ventilation with an endotracheal tube or tracheostomy tube (which bypasses the upper respiratory tract). Even though the upper respiratory tract is not bypassed, additional humidification is still required because of the high-flow rates during noninvasive ventilation (NIV), continuous positive airway pressure (CPAP), or high-flow oxygen treatment. In a bench study by Holland et al., the RH of the NIV circuit (16–26%) was lower than the ambient air RH (27–31%). The incorporation of humidification systems in the NIV circuit had increased RH and AH significantly. However, the evidence on routine humidification during low-flow oxygen treatment is contrasting, owing to the increased risk of bacterial contamination and nosocomial pneumonia, with minimal benefit.

TYPES OF HUMIDIFICATION DEVICES

The choice of humidification system depends on the FiO_2 requirement of the patient, type of oxygen delivery device (high- vs. low-flow system), type of respiratory support (invasive or NIV), type of respiratory failure (risk of hypercapnia), type of interface used for providing NIV (helmet or face or nasal masks), duration of oxygen therapy (short-term or long-term use), and cost of the equipment.

Bubble Humidifier or Cold-water Humidifier

Bubble humidifier (BH) works by vaporizing the gas while passing through nonheated water reservoir. BH is simple and inexpensive. The humidification by BH depends on the surface area of bubbles available for gas vaporization, the ambient room temperature, and the flow rate of gas delivered. The higher the flow rate, the better the humidification. Franchini et al., in their randomized study of long-term nasal low-flow oxygen (NLFO), delivered either by bubble humidifier or without humidification, found that BH did not adequately humidify NLFO, prevent mucociliary dysfunction, or improve airway mucosal hydration. In another study comparing BH versus dry oxygen by Poiroux et al., dry oxygen was noninferior (patient discomfort) to BH for flow rates <4 L/min. A subsequent meta-analysis by Wen et al., also found that routine humidification of low-flow oxygen is not required, considering no significant difference in patient discomfort rates (between humidified oxygen and nonhumidified oxygen), and decreased risk of bacterial contamination with nonhumidified oxygen. Based on this evidence, humidification is not recommended for low-flow oxygen therapy by the German S3 guidelines.

Heat and Moisture Exchanger Filter

The heat and moisture exchanger (HME) filters retain the heat and moisture of expired air that is then returned to patient during inspiration. These are simple (do not require electric circuit to heat), inexpensive, have decreased risk of circuit condensation, and are used commonly in patients receiving invasive or NIV. HME gets blocked by the water or secretions retained and needs frequent (daily) replacement. HME also increases the dead-space ventilation, can cause CO_2 retention, and increase work of breathing. These factors limit the use of HME in subjects with hypercapnic respiratory failure. In the presence of air leaks, the filter recovers less heat and moisture during expiration, thereby decreasing the AH of inspired air. Leaks are more with face masks than nasal masks and with mouth breathing during NIV.

Heated Humidifiers

The heated humidifier (HH) has a heated (by a heated wire) water reservoir that humidies and warms the gases while passing through or over the surface of the water. These are commonly used in patients on high-flow nasal cannula (HFNC) or those being mechanically ventilated (invasive or NIV). Chanques et al., found that HH provides more humidity and better patient comfort rates than BH in patients with high-flow oxygen. Lellouche et al., reported that HH and HME had similar performance (AH between 25 and 30 mgH$_2$O/L), however, with reduced effectiveness of HME in the presence of leaks (15 mgH$_2$O/L). If the ambient air and ventilator output temperatures are high, the humidification by HH is reduced. HH is preferred to HME in patients with hypercapnic respiratory failure, owing to less dead space ventilation. However, using HH increases the risk of circuit condensation.

Different types of HH are available. HHs are expensive compared to BH and HME. Different brands of HH were evaluated in a study by Plotnikow et al., to evaluate their performance (AH and RH) during HFNC therapy with conventional (30-60 L/min) and unconventional flows and seven different heater-wire circuits. Different HHs were found to have variable performances according to the flow rates and circuits used for heating during high-flow oxygenation through a nasal cannula. The highest AH (40.8 mg/L) was achieved with Fisher & Paykel MR850 HH and Medtronic-DAR circuit at a flow of 50 L/min. In comparison while the lowest AH (11.4 mg/L) was recorded with Flexicare FL9000 HH and its own circuit at a flow of 100 L/min. For flows >50 L/min, AH was better with Fisher & Paykel MR850 HH, independent of the type of circuit. Hence, caution is required before selecting the type of HH, heated wire, and flow rates.

RISKS OF HUMIDIFICATION

The commonly observed problems with different types of humidification are: (1) excess water content in the humidifier and spillage into the connecting pipes; (2) high temperature of the humidifier can cause a burning sensation in the upper respiratory tract; (3) blockage of HME filter with water or expelled secretions requiring frequent replacement; and (4) bacterial contamination and infection. The humidifier's water reservoir is an ideal environment for bacteria to grow, especially when heated. Fauci et al., evaluated the safety of reusable humidifiers. The authors found high rates of microbial contamination with reusable oxygen humidifiers (83% in the medical ward, 77% in the surgical ward, and 50% in the emergency area) than with disposable humidifiers (no contamination). *Pseudomonas aeruginosa* and *Staphylococcus aureus* were the most common organisms isolated from the reusable humidifiers. Every effort must be made to avoid such contamination of reservoirs.

To conclude, additional humidification during oxygen therapy is not required in every patient. HH is preferred over other methods of humidification, especially in those being mechanically ventilated and those receiving high-flow nasal oxygen (HFNO). Care should be taken to avoid microbial contamination of reusable humidifier reservoirs.

SUGGESTED READING

1. Franchini ML, Athanazio R, Amato-Lourenço LF, Carreirão-Neto W, Saldiva PH, Lorenzi-Filho G, et al. Oxygen with cold bubble humidification is no better than dry oxygen in preventing mucus dehydration, decreased mucociliary clearance, and decline in pulmonary function. Chest. 2016;150(2):407-14.
2. Gottlieb J, Capetian P, Hamsen U, Janssens U, Karagiannidis C, Kluge S, et al. German S3 guideline: oxygen therapy in the acute care of adult patients. Respiration. 2022;101(2):214-52.

3. La Fauci V, Costa GB, Facciolà A, Conti A, Riso R, Squeri R. Humidifiers for oxygen therapy: what risk for reusable and disposable devices? J Prev Med Hyg. 2017;58(2):E161-E165.
4. Lellouche F, Maggiore SM, Lyazidi A, Deye N, Taillé S, Brochard L. Water content of delivered gases during non-invasive ventilation in healthy subjects. Intensive Care Med. 2009;35(6):987-95.
5. Plotnikow GA, Villalba D, Gogniat E, Quiroga C, Pérez Calvo E, Scapellato JL. Performance of different active humidification systems in high-flow oxygen therapy. Respir Care. 2020;65(9):1250-7.
6. Poiroux L, Piquilloud L, Seegers V, Le Roy C, Colonval K, Agasse C, et al. Effect on comfort of administering bubble-humidified or dry oxygen: the Oxyrea non-inferiority randomized study. Ann Intensive Care. 2018;8(1):126.
7. Rodriguez AME, Scala R, Soroksky A, BaHammam A, de Klerk A, Valipour A, et al. Clinical review: humidifiers during non-invasive ventilation—key topics and practical implications. Crit Care. 2012;16(1):203.
8. Wen Z, Wang W, Zhang H, Wu C, Ding J, Shen M. Is humidified better than non-humidified low-flow oxygen therapy? A systematic review and meta-analysis. J Adv Nurs. 2017;73(11):2522-33.

High-Flow Nasal Cannula

CHAPTER 18

Harjit Dumra, Mansi Dandnaik

INTRODUCTION

The most commonly prescribed intervention for any patient in respiratory distress is the supplemental oxygen. Conventional delivery devices usually deliver oxygen at flows <15 L/min and many a time with associated problems primarily dryness and irritation of the airway. In patients with respiratory failure the inspiratory flow requirements varies from 30 L/min to occasionally even >100 L/min. This leads to a substantial difference between delivered and required inspiratory flow ultimately resulting in an FiO_2 which is both lower than expected and often inconstant. While use of noninvasive ventilation (NIV) might overcome some of these challenges, it is often associated with ineffective synchrony and poor patient compliance, the high-flow nasal cannula (HFNC) is designed to overcome most of the aforementioned limitations of the presently available oxygen delivery devices and the previously available robust evidence for its effective use is now consolidated by the remarkable improvement in availability and experience with the device during the COVID-19 pandemic.

While many of the initial studies were in the neonatal population, we now have clinical trials showing significant benefits in the adult populations as well. In the literature, various terms have been coined for this method of oxygen delivery—the commonly used being nasal high-flow ventilation, mini-continuous positive airway pressure (CPAP), nasal high flow, transnasal insufflation, HFNC oxygen therapy, etc. Here, we intend to use the term HFNC throughout the text.

OBJECTIVE

The air/oxygen blender in the HFNC can generate a total flow of up to 60–80 L/min and FiO_2 between 21 and 100% irrespective of flow rates. The gas mixture is humidified and heated from 31 to 37°C prior to being delivered. To minimize condensation, the gas is delivered through wide-bore nasal prongs and heated tubing. **Figure 1** shows basic structure of the HFNC and the interface.

PHYSIOLOGICAL EFFECTS

High flow of adequately humidified and heated gas is considered to have a significant physiological effects. Currently, established mechanisms are believed to be the reason for efficacy HFNC and include:

- High flow washes out carbon dioxide (CO_2) in physiological dead space.
- HFNC improves thoracoabdominal synchrony compared to face mask. It reduces dead space and washes out CO_2. Itagaki et al. found that HFNC reduces breathing frequency but arterial carbon dioxide level ($PaCO_2$) and tidal volume (VT) remains constant. This provide

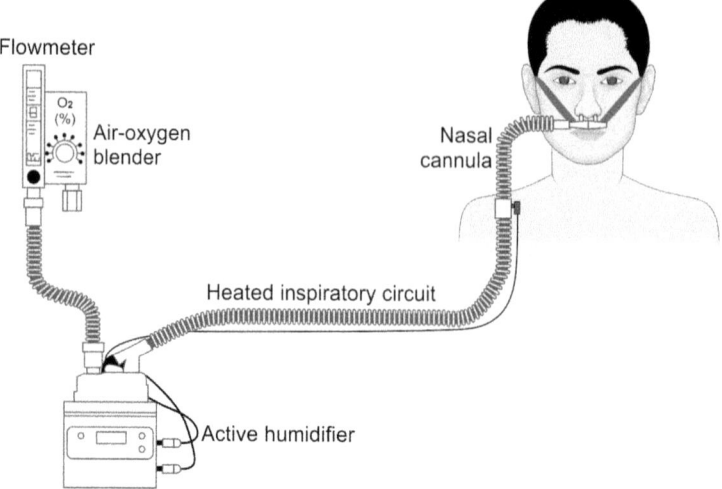

Fig. 1: Principle setup of high-flow nasal cannula oxygen therapy. An air/oxygen blender, allowing from 0.21 to 1.0 FiO$_2$, generates up to 60 L/min flow. The gas is heated and humidified through an active heated humidifier and delivered via a single-limb heated inspiratory circuit. The patient breaths the adequately heated and humidified medical gas through nasal cannulas with a large diameter.

indirect proof that HFNC reduces minute ventilation by reduction in dead space.

- *Positive end-expiratory pressure (PEEP):* Even though it is an open system, the flow of HFNC against the resistance of expiratory flow increases airway pressure. With the mouth closed, increasing inspiratory flow leads to increased mean airway pressure with mouth closed. This observation is validated by numerous studies. Parke et al. compared HFNC with face mask delivery in postcardiac surgery patients. Even 35 L/min flow could generate PEEP of 2.7 ± 1.04 cmH$_2$O with closed mouth and 1.2 ± 0.76 cmH$_2$O with open mouth. There is no positive pressure when the same flow given with the face mask. In postoperative patients when inspiratory flow was increased at 40, 50, and 60 L/min, airway pressure increased by 1.52 ± 0.7, 2.21 ± 0.8, and 3.1 ± 1.2 cmH$_2$O, respectively. While the increased airway pressure is relatively low compared to closed ventilation systems, it is still adequate enough to increase lung volume and recruit collapsed alveoli.
- *Increased end-expiratory volume and decreased respiratory rate:* Increased pharyngeal pressure by HFNC generates PEEP but it was unclear initially whether HFNC actually recruits collapsed alveoli and increases lung volume. Corley et al. used electrical lung impedance tomography to evaluate end-expiratory lung volume and found it was more with HFNC than low flow oxygen therapy. Similarly, Riera et al. measured end-expiratory lung volume in supine and in prone postures, by electrical lung impedance tomography. It was more with HFNC in both positions. These all causes improved lung mechanics resulting in decreased respiratory rate. These improvement in lung mechanics ultimately result in decreased respiratory rate.

- *Humidification:* Because gas is generally warmed to 37°C and completely humidified, mucociliary functions remain good and little discomfort is reported.

INDICATIONS

- *Hypoxic respiratory failure:* Acute hypoxemic respiratory failure (AHRF) occurs due to airspace collapse due to exudates related to pneumonia, pulmonary edema, or hemorrhage leading to intrapulmonary shunting of blood. PEEP provided by HFNC makes it a much more effective option than low-flow oxygen devices in this setting. The FLORALI (Flow Nasal Oxygen Therapy in Resuscitation of Patients with Acute Lung Injury) trial found that use of HFNC is associated with reduced intensive care unit (ICU) and 90-day mortality although it did not reduce intubation rate among hypoxic immune-competent patients. The results also suggested increased degree of comfort, decreased respiratory rate, less dyspnea severity, increased ventilator-free days without any adverse effect related to HFNC. The trial was underpowered for the primary outcome which was intubation rate. It was not replicated by two subsequent randomized controlled trials. However, later studies by Stephen et al. and Maggiore et al. showed NIV and HFNC to be equally efficient as in avoiding intubation and reducing mortality. HFNC is definitely more comfortable alternative for the patients struggling or not tolerating NIV under close observation. The decision of initiating and continuing patients on HFNC requires objective variables to predict success. Using ROX (respiratory rate and oxygenation) index is studied variable for the same. Roca et al. introduced the concept of using ratio of SpO_2/FiO_2 to breathing frequency, known as the ROX index. This index that combines oxygenation and breathing frequency to predict the need to switch from HFNC to mechanical ventilation. The cut-off value of the ROX index after 12 hour of HFNC was 4.88. This suggests that once patient is on HFNC for more than 12 hours and ROX index >4.88 success possibility is high. Later on with larger multicenter trial, they explored the cut-off values for ROX to predict HFNC failure. HFNC failure was expected at 2, 6, and 12 hours if the ROX index was >2.85, 3.47, or 3.85, respectively. An important consideration is HFNC gas flow affects the ROX index. Mauri et al. studied that when gas flow was modified from 30 to 60 L/min in majority (70%) of the ROX indexes increased while the nonsignificant change in the remaining subjects. The same ROX index can be used with regard to liberation and weaning from HFNC. Rodriguez et al. investigated in retrospective study noticed that the ROX index to predict successful separation 88% of subjects at the first attempt, and FiO_2 <0.4 and ROX >9.2 were predictive of HFNC separation success.
- *Hypercapnic respiratory failure:* NIV is time-tested intervention as far as treating chronic obstructive pulmonary disease (COPD) exacerbation or other hypercapnic failure in the acute setting. However, the low level of patient comfort and compliance is troublesome for NIV. Dzira et al. discovered that in COPD GOLD stage III and IV patients, HFNC at flow rates >30 L/min decreased the diaphragmatic work of breathing, respiratory rate, inspiratory time to total breath time ratio comparable to NIV. Recently published meta-analyses indicated that compared with NIV, HFNC could significantly reduce $PaCO_2$ level, the

incidence of nasal facial skin breakdown, and length of hospital stay. Additionally, there was no significant differences between the two groups in incidence of tracheal intubation, PaO_2, and mortality.

- *Postextubation:* Reintubation is associated with increased ICU and in-hospital length of stay and mortality. HFNC was used in different postsurgical setting particularly postcardiac and abdominal surgeries and results are encouraging. Hernandez and colleagues published two seminal papers in JAMA regarding the use of HFNC in low- and high-risk postextubation patients. They concluded that in low-risk patients postextubation HFNC was superior to standard care. In the high-risk patients, HFNC was noninferior to noninvasive mechanical ventilation. Furthermore, strategy of combining NIV with HFNC in high-risk patients was superior to all other modalities.
- *Sleep apnea:* HFNC is kind of CPAP device is associated with reduced apnea–hypopnea index and arousals in adults. McGinley et al. confirmed that HFNC when used for obstructive sleep apnea alleviated upper airway obstruction. Acute stroke can lead to sleep-disordered breathing in sleep and is associated with poor neurological and overall outcome. They poorly tolerate CPAP because of discomfort. HFNC with the flow 18 L/min not only well tolerated but also lead to decreased oxygen desaturation index and the apnea–hypopnea index. This makes HFNC a viable alternative for acute stroke patients.
- *Preoxygenation:* Preoxygenating every patient before intubation is mandatory. HFNC therapy can achieve high PO_2 by very high-flow rates and high FiO_2 even in an alert awake patient. This gives enough time for intubation process before patient desaturates. Historically, for awake patients preoxygenation is performed with a nonrebreather mask (NRBM). However, Miguel-Mantanes et al. found that HFNC significantly improves oxygenation during intubation compared NRBM. While in one retrospective analysis, Besnier and Emmanuel et al. found that NIV such as bilevel positive airway pressure (BiPAP) yields similar results to HFNC with better compliance. This suggests that HFNC therapy is superior to NRBM and noninferior to NIV for preoxygenation.
- *Do not intubate the patient:* Patients in palliative care or immunocompromised, where invasive ventilator support is associated with increased risk of infection, HFNC therapy is a viable alternative. A meta-analysis and review by Hui-Bin Huang et al. explored HFNC therapy in immunocompromised patients with acute respiratory failure. They compared HFNC to both low-flow nasal cannula and NIV and HFNC found reduce both intubation rate and mortality in the immunocompromised.
- *Emergency department:* Patients presenting with dyspnea and/or hypoxemia on emergency room entry had faster symptomatic relief and improved oxygenation when HFNC was used upfront instead of conventional oxygen. Nuttapol et al. confirmed the same in prospective randomized comparative study.
- *Others:* HFNC can be used as an aid to difficult bronchoscopies. Lucangelo et al. in a study compared bronchoscopies in adults with HFNC at two different flows: 40 and 60 L/min flow and compared it with 40 L/min flow with venturi mask. At the end of the procedure, 60 L/min resulted with better oxygenation compared to 40 L/min with both the methods.

ISSUES OF CONCERN

High-flow nasal cannula like many other medical interventions is not without drawbacks and limitations. When we compare it with low-flow oxygen therapy systems, HFNC is expensive, more complex requiring training to initiate care, high oxygen consumption, decreased mobility, a potential to delay intubation, and might inappropriately delay of end-of-life decisions. Furthermore, limitations and potential risk factors to NIV apply to some extent with HFNC. That includes patients who are not ideal candidates are those with hemodynamic instability, alteration of consciousness, excessive secretion, facial injury, those with bulbar weakness with the risk of aspiration.

CONCLUSION

High-flow nasal cannula oxygen delivery has been gaining attention as a well-tolerated and simple alternative of respiratory support in critically ill patients particularly with hypoxic respiratory failure. Though HFNC has been used for a wide variety of indications particularly in the post-COVID era. We still need more rigorous evidence for newer indications, criteria for initiation, treatment escalation, and discontinuation.

SUGGESTED READING

1. Besnier E, Guernon K, Bubenheim M, Gouin P, Carpentier D, Béduneau G, et al. Pre-oxygenation with high-flow nasal cannula oxygen therapy and non-invasive ventilation for intubation in the intensive care unit. Intensive Care Med. 2016;42(8):1291-2.
2. Corley A, Caruana LR, Barnett AG, Tronstad O, Fraser JF. Oxygen delivery through high-flow nasal cannulae increase end-expiratory lung volume and reduce respiratory rate in post-cardiac surgical patients. Br J Anaesth. 2011;107(6):998-1004.
3. Frat JP, Thille AW, Mercat A, Girault C, Ragot S, Perbet S, et al.; FLORALI Study Group; REVA Network. High-flow oxygen through nasal cannula in acute hypoxemic respiratory failure. N Engl J Med. 2015;372(23):2185-96.
4. Haba-Rubio J, Andries D, Rey V, Michel P, Tafti M, Heinzer R. Effect of transnasal insufflation on sleep disordered breathing in acute stroke: a preliminary study. Sleep Breath. 2012;16:759-64.
5. Hernández G, Vaquero C, Colinas L, Cuena R, González P, Canabal A, et al. Effect of postextubation high-flow nasal cannula vs. noninvasive ventilation on reintubation and postextubation respiratory failure in high-risk patients: a randomized clinical trial. JAMA. 2016;316(15):1565-74.
6. Hernández G, Vaquero C, González P, Subira C, Frutos-Vivar F, Rialp G, et al. Effect of postextubation high-flow nasal cannula vs. conventional oxygen therapy on reintubation in low-risk patients: a randomized clinical trial. JAMA. 2016;315(13):1354-61.
7. Huang HB, Peng JM, Weng L, Liu GY, Du B. High-flow oxygen therapy in immunocompromised patients with acute respiratory failure: a review and meta-analysis. J Crit Care. 2018;43:300-5.
8. Itagaki T, Okuda N, Tsunano Y, Kohata H, Nakataki E, Onodera M, et al. Effect of high-flow nasal cannula on thoraco-abdominal synchrony in adult critically ill patients. Respir Care. 2014;59:70-4.
9. Lucangelo U, Vassallo FG, Marras E, Ferluga M, Beziza E, Comuzzi L, et al. High-flow nasal interface improves oxygenation in patients undergoing bronchoscopy. Crit Care Res Pract. 2012;2012:506382.
10. Maggiore SM, Idone FA, Vaschetto R, Festa R, Cataldo A, Antonicelli F, et al. Nasal high-flow versus Venturi mask oxygen therapy after extubation. Effects on oxygenation, comfort, and clinical outcome. Am J Respir Crit Care Med. 2014;190(3):282-8.
11. Mauri T, Carlesso E, Spinelli E, Turrini C, Corte FD, Russo R, et al. Increasing support by nasal high flow acutely modifies the ROX index in hypoxemic patients: a physiologic study. J Crit Care. 2019;53:183-5.

12. Miguel-Montanes R, Hajage D, Messika J, Bertrand F, Gaudry S, Rafat C, et al. Use of high-flow nasal cannula oxygen therapy to prevent desaturation during tracheal intubation of intensive care patients with mild-to-moderate hypoxemia. Crit Care Med. 2015;43(3):574-83.
13. Nihimura M. High-flow nasal cannula oxygen therapy in adults. J Intensive Care. 2015;3(1):15.
14. Parke R, McGunness S, Eccleston M. Nasal high-flow therapy delivers low level positive airway pressure. Br J Anaesth. 2009;103:886-90.
15. Riera J, Pérez P, Cortés J, Roca O, Masclans JR, Rello J. Effect of high-flow nasal cannula and body position on end-expiratory lung volume: a cohort study using electrical impedance tomography. Respir Care. 2013;58:589-96.
16. Ritchie JE, Williams AB, Gerard C, Hockey H. Evaluation of a humidified nasal high-flow oxygen system, using oxygraphy, capnography and measurement of upper airway pressures. Anaesth Intensive Care. 2011;39:1103-1.
17. Rittayamai N, Tscheikuna J, Praphruetkit N, Kijpinyochai S. Use of high-flow nasal cannula for acute dyspnea and hypoxemia in the emergency department. Respir Care. 2015;60(10):1377-82.
18. Roca O, Caralt B, Messika J, Samper M, Sztrymf B, Hernández G, et al. An index combining respiratory rate and oxygenation to predict outcome of nasal high-flow therapy. Am J Respir Crit Care Med. 2019;199(11):1368-76.
19. Roca O, Messika J, Caralt B, Garćıa-de-Acilu M, Sztrymf B, Ricard JD, et al. Predicting success of high-flow nasal cannula in pneumonia patients with hypoxemic respiratory failure: the utility of the ROX index. J Crit Care. 2016;35:200-5.
20. Roca O, Riera J, Torres F, Masclans JR. High-flow oxygen therapy in acute respiratory failure. Respir Care. 2010;55:408-13.
21. Rodriguez M, Thille AW, Boissier F, Veinstein A, Chatellier D, Robert R, et al. Predictors of successful separation from high-flow nasal oxygen therapy in patients with acute respiratory failure: a retrospective monocenter study. Ann Intensive Care. 2019;9(1):101.
22. Sharma S, Danckers M, Sanghavi D, Chakraborty RK. (2022). High flow nasal cannula. [online] In: StatPearls [Internet]. Treasure Island (FL): StatPearls Publishing.
23. Stéphan F, Bérard L, Rézaiguia-Delclaux S, Amaru P; BiPOP Study Group. High-flow nasal cannula therapy versus intermittent noninvasive ventilation in obese subjects after cardiothoracic surgery. Respir Care. 2017;62(9):1193-202.
24. Sztrymf B, Messika J, Bertrand F, Hurel D, Leon R, Dreyfuss D, et al. Beneficial effects of humidified high flow nasal oxygen in critical care patients: a prospective pilot study. Intensive Care Med. 2011;37:1780-6.
25. Thille AW, Muller G, Gacouin A, Coudroy R, Decavèle M, Sonneville R, et al. Effect of postextubation high-flow nasal oxygen with noninvasive ventilation vs. high-flow nasal oxygen alone on reintubation among patients at high risk of extubation failure: a randomized clinical trial. JAMA. 2019;322(15):1465-75.
26. Xu Z, Zhu L, Zhan J, Liu L. The efficacy and safety of high-flow nasal cannula therapy in patients with COPD and type II respiratory failure: a meta-analysis and systematic review. Eur J Med Res. 2021;26(1):122.

Hyperbaric Oxygen Therapy

CHAPTER 19

Gunjan Chanchalani, Sunil Amin, Kanwalpreet Sodhi

INTRODUCTION

Hyperbaric oxygen therapy (HBOT) involves placing a patient inside a chamber which is pressurized to >1 (up to 3) atmospheric pressure, with 100% oxygen. This exposure has shown to produce many physiological effects in the body tissues, apart from increased plasma oxygen concentration. Today, HBOT is being used for varied indications, including many acute pathologies, as well as for chronic long-term illnesses.

HISTORY

Use of HBOT for a variety of medical conditions, dates back to the late 1600s. Its initial use was mainly for divers and "the bends", however after the work of Ita Boerema and his colleagues in the 20th century, its use expanded. Studies were later conducted by various groups, to understand the safety limits of the barometric pressure and oxygen, and its duration. Currently, HBOT is approved for various acute and chronic conditions and concise, evidence-based guidelines are available for its safe use.

METHOD OF ADMINISTRATION

Equipment Needed

Pressurized Chambers

- Monoplace chambers **(Fig. 1):** Single occupancy chamber or monoplace chamber is usually used for treatment

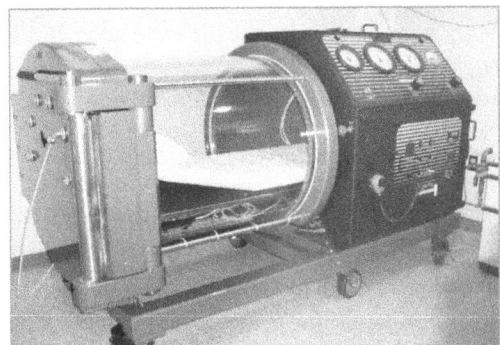

Fig. 1: Monoplace hyperbaric chamber.
Source: https://www.hyperbaricstore.com/product/hypertec-hybrid-3200/ [Last accessed June, 2022].

of chronic conditions, with stable vitals. It is a long tube and the patient lies inside it. A single patient inside the chamber breathes pressurized 100% oxygen.

- Multiplace **(Fig. 2):** These chambers can hold multiple patients at one time. Patients on ventilator or those needing special equipment are usually placed in a multiplace chambers, which can even hold an overseeing physician. The chamber is pressurized with air, and the patients individually breathe 100% oxygen via a face mask, oxygen hood, or an endotracheal tube.

Technique

A single session of hyperbaric therapy is administered for a duration of 45 minutes to 5 hours, with pressures of 2.5–3 atm

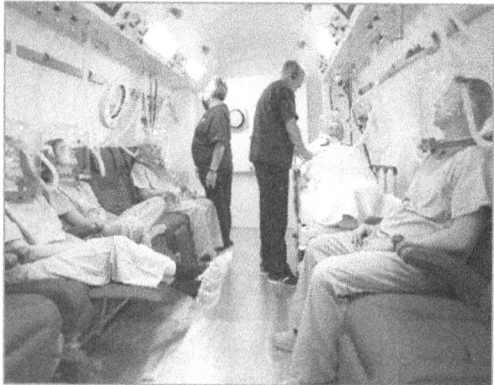

Fig. 2: Multiplace hyperbaric chamber.
Source: https://www.medicalexpo.com/prod/hyperbaric-modular-systems/product-78313-479201.html [Last accessed June, 2022].

with 100% oxygen, based on the medical indication. Heliox (helium/oxygen) or nitrox (nitrogen/oxygen mix) may be used in cases of decompression illness. The number of sessions vary—needing one to two treatment sessions in an acute therapy and up to 60 treatment sessions in chronic conditions.

Safety Regulations

Each chamber has strict regulations, frequent inspections, and specifications. Keen vigilance of the staff helps avoid catastrophic events like failure of the chamber and fire. No combustible material (oil, electronics, or other nonapproved items) is allowed inside the chamber. Patients are grounded to avoid any static sparks.

MECHANISM OF ACTION OF HYPERBARIC OXYGEN THERAPY

Benefits of HBOT are mainly secondary to simple physics of increased oxygen tension in the tissues.
- *Increased delivery of oxygen:* Henry's law states that the amount of an ideal gas dissolved in solution is directly proportional to its partial pressure. At room ambient atmospheric pressure (1.0 atm, 21% FiO_2), the dissolved oxygen concentration in the plasma is 0.3 mL/dL, which increases to 1.5 mL/dL upon inhaling pure oxygen (1.0 atm, 100% FiO_2). Upon administering HBOT at 3.0 atm the dissolved plasma oxygen content increases to 6 mL/dL. This dissolved oxygen content is adequate to meet the resting oxygen requirements of the tissues, irrespective of the adequacy of the hemoglobin-bound oxygen content. Thus, use of HBOT has improved tissue survival in cases of profound anemia, ischemia of the tissues, and carbon monoxide (CO) poisoning.
- *Gas bubble size reduction:* Boyle's law states that pressure is inversely proportional to the volume. So HBOT helps reduce the volume of the nitrogen bubbles by increasing the pressure exerted on it. This principle explains the role of HBOT in decompression illness. The bubble volume has been found to decrease by approximately two-thirds, at a pressure of 3.0 atm. The decrease in bubble size is further augmented by the replacement of the inert nitrogen inside the bubbles with oxygen, which can be rapidly metabolized by the tissues.
- *Carbon monoxide antagonism:* Carbon monoxide has a 200–250 times higher affinity for hemoglobin than oxygen, forming carboxyhemoglobin (COHb) and thus reducing the oxygen carrying capacity of the blood. Carboxyhemoglobin further causes a leftward shift of the oxyhemoglobin curve and impairs the oxygen release at the tissue level. The half-life of COHb is 4–6 hours at room air, which drops to 40–80 minutes on breathing 100% oxygen at ambient pressure, further decreasing it to 15–30 minutes with HBOT.

- *Improved wound healing:* HBOT modulates the inflammatory process in the injured and ischemic tissues via increased production of reactive oxygen species (free radicals, hydrogen peroxide, hypochlorous acid) and nitric oxide. This increased oxidative stress reduces vasogenic edema, induces tissue vasoconstriction, facilitates angiogenesis, fibroblast formation, and wound healing. It also ameliorates ischemia–reperfusion-induced leukocyte influx, augments neutrophil bactericidal activity, kills anaerobes (*Clostridium perfringens*), and inhibits growth of other pathogens. It also neutralizes the alpha toxins produced by *Clostridium* species.
- *Other effects:* HBOT potentiates the effect of some antibiotics like aminoglycosides and quinolones.

INDICATIONS

Approved Indications

There are 14 conditions approved by the Undersea and Hyperbaric Medical Society for HBOT, including:

1. *Decompression sickness/"the bends":* HBOT accelerates diffusion of gas bubbles into the surrounding tissue, immediate reduction in the bubble volume, improved oxygenation of ischemic tissues, and cerebral edema reduction.
2. *Acute gas/air emboli—venous/arterial:* Use of HBOT in vascular gas/air emboli helps decrease the size of emboli, facilitates the removal of gas bubbles by the lungs, and decreases reperfusion injury.
3. *Necrotizing fasciitis:* HBOT is an adjunct to surgical debridement, antibiotics, and good critical care practices. HBOT helps the diffusion of oxygen to the ischemic tissues, improves oxygenation to the ischemic tissues, reduces hypoxic leucocyte dysfunction, thus eventually reducing the progression and spread of infection.
4. *Gas gangrene/Clostridium myonecrosis:* HBOT up to three atmospheric pressure, helps to increase the tissue O_2 pressure above 300 mm Hg, which helps stop alpha toxin production and inhibits bacterial growth. HBOT in gas gangrene has been found to be life- and limb-saving.
5. *Refractory osteomyelitis:* HBOT for up to 4-6 weeks may be required in cases of refractory osteomyelitis. It should be administered as an adjunct to surgical debridement and culture-directed antibiotics and sessions should begin soon after surgical intervention.
6. *Severe, acute blood loss anemia:* Pulsed HBOT helps correct the accumulating oxygen debt due to compromised oxygen delivery from severe anemia, when transfusion is not possible.
7. *Failed/compromised skin grafts and flaps:* Useful in flaps and grafts compromised by irradiation and decreased perfusion or hypoxia.
8. *Chronic/delayed radiation injury:* HBOT reduces soft tissue and bony necrosis and fibrosis secondary to radiation, by inducing neovascularization in the hypoxic tissues. Also HBOT is likely to stimulate and mobilize the stem cells in the irradiated tissue.
9. *Carbon monoxide poisoning:* HBOT hastens dissociation of COHb, faster than breathing 100% oxygen at sea-level pressure. Animal studies have shown benefit of HBOT in reducing central nervous system (CNS) injuries, hastening cardiovascular recovery, and decreased mortality in CO poisoning. The mechanism includes an improvement in mitochondrial oxidation, lipid peroxidation inhibition, and inhibition of adhesion of leucocytes to injured microvasculature.

In cases of cyanide poisoning with CO toxicity, HBOT has been recommended as an adjunct therapy.

10. *Acute thermal injury:* Adjunctive HBOT helps modulate the inflammatory process in burn injuries, thus decreasing edema formation, decreasing the progression of the depth of the thermal injury, preserving marginally viable tissue, enhancing host defenses, and promoting wound closure.
11. *Compartment syndromes/compression injury/crush injury:* HBOT helps improve oxygen availability to hypoxic tissues with inadequate perfusion in the immediate postinjury period. The availability of improved tissue oxygen tensions after HBOT helps to maintain cellular metabolic functions and improves wound healing, angiogenesis, and mitigates reperfusion injury.
12. *Intracranial abscess:* HBOT helps by inhibiting the predominant anaerobic flora in the abscess, causes a decrease in the perifocal brain edema, helps enhance the host defense mechanisms, and also helps in concomitant skull osteomyelitis.
13. *Arterial insufficiency:* In the management of central retinal artery occlusion, HBOT has shown to produce an improvement in vision, if administered in the first 24 hours of symptoms.
    In the treatment of ischemic, infected diabetic foot ulcers, HBOT helps maximize oxygen delivery, neovascularization, and thus increases wound blood flow and healing.
14. *Idiopathic acute sensory hearing loss:* Used within 2 weeks of symptom onset, HBOT significantly improved hearing in studies.

Off-label Indications

Hyperbaric oxygen therapy has been used for various off-label indications like stroke, autism, and attention deficit hyperactivity disorder (ADHD).

Its role in mild traumatic brain injury, post-traumatic stress injury remains controversial, however under licensed experienced hands, it can be used as an alternative treatment when primary treatment has failed to show a benefit.

Animal Studies

In sepsis, HBOT has shown to have a potential to reduce organ failure in animal studies. Adjunctive use of HBOT in infective endocarditis, may play a role in decreasing morbidity, mortality, and improve the long-term outcomes.

CONTRAINDICATIONS

Absolute Contraindication

Untreated pneumothorax—use of HBOT may worsen the pneumothorax and lead to development of life-threatening tension pneumothorax. A thoracostomy tube should be placed before placing in the hyperbaric chamber.

Relative Contraindications

- Chronic obstructive lung disease—risk of oxygen-induced hypoventilation and increased ventilation/perfusion (V/Q) mismatch, hypercarbia.
- Asymptomatic pulmonary blebs or bullae on chest radiograph, emphysema, asthma, risk of air trapping and progression to pneumothorax.
- Upper respiratory or sinus infections—with associated eustachian tube dysfunction—can lead to barotrauma of the tympanic membrane.
- Recent ear or thoracic surgery, otosclerosis, eye surgery.
- Claustrophobia.

- Use of certain drugs like disulfiram (blocks superoxide dismutase, which protects against oxygen toxicity), cisplatin (can impair wound healing), mafenide acetate (can cause local carbon dioxide production and acidosis), bleomycin (increased risk of interstitial pneumonitis and fibrosis).
- High uncontrolled fever, seizures, oxygen toxicity can decrease seizure threshold.
- Implanted devices such as pacemakers and defibrillators (determine their safety, ability to function in a high-pressure environment, and the risk of triggering a fire inside the chamber).
- Epidural pumps (risk of device malfunction or deformation).
- Pregnancy—HBOT however should be considered in pregnant patients with CO poisoning.
- History of spontaneous pneumothorax.
- Congenital spherocytosis—may trigger hemolysis due to increased partial pressure of oxygen.

COMPLICATIONS

- *Barotrauma:* The most common complication of HBOT is barotrauma, due to expansion of gases inside a confined space. The injury depends on the organ involved:
  - *Ear:* Eardrum rupture, middle ear injuries, leaking fluid
  - *Sinuses:* Sinus barotrauma (sinus squeeze), usually seen in patients with upper respiratory tract infections or allergic rhinitis.
  - *Lung:* Lung collapse, pulmonary edema, pneumothorax
  - Rupture of the small vessels.
- *Oxygen toxicity:*
- *Central nervous system:* Seizures
  - *Eye:* Reversible myopia
- Lowered blood sugar in patients with diabetes mellitus, on insulin
- *Equipment-related:*
  - Chamber failure
  - Fire and explosions
- *Risk to the chamber attendants:*
  - Decompression illness (decompression sickness and arterial gas embolism)
  - Barotrauma (majority barometric otitis)
  - Other health issues—osteonecrosis
  - Death—due to fires.

THE FUTURE

Hyperbaric oxygen therapy has the potential to be useful in many conditions involving the ischemia-reperfusion injury and inflammation. Its use in acute coronary syndrome, including myocardial infarction, the systemic inflammatory response syndrome, traumatic brain or spinal cord injury, sickle cell crisis, frostbite, fibromyalgia, and acute stroke, needs further studies and evaluation.

SUGGESTED READING

1. Bennett MH, Lehm JP, Jepson N. Hyperbaric oxygen therapy for acute coronary syndrome. Cochrane Database Syst Rev. 2015; 2015(7):CD004818.
2. Camporesi EM, Bosco G. Mechanisms of action of hyperbaric oxygen therapy. Undersea Hyperb Med. 2014;41(3):247-52.
3. Dauwe PB, Pulikkottil BJ, Lavery L, Stuzin JM, Rohrich RJ. Does hyperbaric oxygen therapy work in facilitating acute wound healing: a systematic review. Plast Reconstr Surg. 2014;133(2):208e-15e.
4. Dennis TJ, Mohr NM, Bailey OE. The role of hyperbaric oxygen therapy in septic shock: is it time for human studies? Undersea Hyperb Med. 2022;49(1):43-55.
5. Heyboer M 3rd, Sharma D, Santiago W, McCulloch N. Hyperbaric oxygen therapy: side

effects defined and quantified. Adv Wound Care (New Rochelle). 2017;6(6):210-24.
6. Kirby JP, Snyder J, Schuerer DJE, Peters JS, Bochicchio GV. Essentials of hyperbaric oxygen therapy: 2019 review. Mo Med. 2019;116(3):176-9.
7. National Hyperbaric Treatment Center. History of HBOT. [online] Available from https://nationalhyperbaric.com/hyperbaric-oxygen-therapy/history-of-hbot-therapy/#:~:text=The%20Start%20of%20Oxygen%20X Therapy,diving%20full%20for%20underwater%20repair [Last accessed June, 2022].
8. Pougnet R, Pougnet L, Lucas D, Henckes A, Loddé B, Dewitte JD. Health effects of hyperbaric exposure on chamber attendants: a literature review. Int Marit Health. 2018; 69(1):58-62.
9. Rusyniak DE, Kirk MA, May JD, Kao LW, Brizendine EJ, Welch JL, et al. Hyperbaric oxygen therapy in acute ischemic stroke: results of the Hyperbaric Oxygen in Acute Ischemic Stroke Trial Pilot Study. Stroke. 2003;34(2):571-4.
10. Thom SR. Hyperbaric oxygen: its mechanisms and efficacy. Plast Reconstr Surg. 2011; 127(Suppl 1):131S-41S.
11. Undersea and Hyperbaric Medical Society. Indications for hyperbaric oxygen therapy. [online] Available from https://www.uhms.org/resources/hbo-indications.html [Last accessed June, 2022].

Oxygen Toxicity

CHAPTER 20

Shrikant Sahasrabudhe, Beena Daniel

INTRODUCTION

Always remember that oxygen is a drug so use it judiciously. As we know, oxygen is life and it has been present in the atmosphere for 5 billion years. Priestley discovered oxygen and was among the first to suggest that there may be adverse effects of "pure air." Today, oxygen is the most commonly used therapeutic agent in hospitals. The partial pressure of oxygen in inspired air at the sea level is about 160 mm Hg. Hyperoxia is basically a condition wherein oxygen is breathed in at a higher than normal partial pressure and can cause oxygen toxicity. The lower respiratory tract is predominantly affected than the upper airways wherein it can cause damage to alveolar walls, including fibrosis. The clinical settings in which oxygen toxicity occurs is predominantly divided into two groups:

1. *Acute:* It is also called the "Bert" effect. This is a condition in which the patient is exposed to very high concentrations of oxygen for a short duration and mainly has central nervous system (CNS) manifestations.
2. *Chronic:* It is also called the "Smith" effect. This is a condition in which the patient is exposed to lower concentrations of oxygen for a longer duration and mainly has pulmonary effects. Severe cases of oxygen toxicity can lead to cell damage and death.

BACKGROUND

In a few of the prospective studies, it has been documented that in normal volunteers and patients on ventilator exposure to 100% oxygen for at least 24 hours is "safe". But contrary to these findings, it has also been documented that such exposure of oxygen can cause damage to the lower respiratory tract and is responsible for decrease in vital capacity and diffusing lung capacity, which raised concerns about the time and dose of oxygen. In a study published way back in the year 1983, it has been clearly shown that normal subjects exposed to 95% oxygen for as short as 17 hours developed reversible alveolar capillary leak and patients exposed to higher oxygen concentration (100%) for 2–3 days may develop permanent pulmonary structural derangements, leading to parenchymal lung injury and lung fibrosis.

PATHOPHYSIOLOGY

Oxygen delivery depends upon oxygen saturation which in turn depends upon oxygen supplementation. It will increase oxygen saturation in patients who are hyperemic. Oxygen-derived free radicals is the basic etiological factor in the development of these toxic effects. Free radicals are generated due to the mitochondrial oxido-reductive processes and are also induced by the function of enzymes such as xanthine/urate oxidase at extramitochondrial sites, from auto-oxidative reactions, and by phagocytes during the bacterial killing. Free radicals, in turn, are responsible for lipid peroxidation, especially in the cell membranes; they also subdue nucleic acids and protein synthesis and modify cellular enzymes **(Fig. 1A)**. During the ensuing of the hyperoxic process, a large influx of reactive oxygen species (ROS) is produced. ROS overproduction, caused by oxygen overexposure, disrupts the balance between oxidants and antioxidants and results in damage to cells and tissues **(Fig. 1B)**. Oxygen is toxic to the lungs when high fraction of inspired oxygen (FiO_2 >0.60) is administered over an extended exposure time (≥24 hours) at normal barometric pressure, i.e., atmospheric absolute air (1 ATA).

It can also exert nonradical-mediated injury by altering cellular metabolism or by hyperoxia-induced glutamic acid decarboxylase inhibition in CNS. Also, reduced levels of gamma-amino butyric acid (GABA) are seen concomitantly with the occurrence of seizures. Animal studies have revealed gray matter and neuronal necrosis with a single, short exposure producing ultrastructural changes in the anterior horn gray matter, and severe prolonged exposure causing hemorrhagic necrosis in the brain at selective sites. In the lungs, there is a marked exudation with congestion. This is sometimes associated with intra-alveolar hemorrhages, necrosis of the alveolar cells, and epithelial desquamation along with initial damage at the level of capillary endothelium, which is followed by edematous thickening of alveolar septum, destruction of type 1 pneumocytes, formation of hyaline membranes, intra-alveolar hemorrhages, and areas of atelectasis.

CLINICAL PRESENTATION OF HYPEROXIC ACUTE LUNG INJURY

As we are aware, acute respiratory distress syndrome (ARDS) can be of pulmonary or extrapulmonary pathology but the condition which is exacerbated by hyperoxia mimics ARDS and is called hyperoxic acute lung injury (HALI). As in ARDS, there is systemic release of pro-inflammatory cytokines along with mast cells, which affect lung vasculature. It culminates into the activation of macrophages and recruits neutrophils, leukotrienes, oxidants, and platelet-activating factor, and the cascade continues **(Table 1)**.

EVALUATION/DIAGNOSIS

A high index of suspicion is the key to suspect oxygen toxicity in a patient who is on high FiO_2 for a longer period of time. In an intensive care unit (ICU), ARDS is the common clinical setting when one can suspect or expect oxygen toxicity. We need to monitor oxygen saturation regularly which is very commonly done. Witnessing elevated work of breathing can be an early sign of oxygen toxicity. Performing pulmonary function test (PFT) is not feasible in ICU but can be a possibility in non-ICU patients, mainly to look for features suggestive of restrictive lung pathology. Getting a bedside *chest X-ray* which can reveal alveolo-interstitial shadows and in the 21st century extensive use of bedside *lung ultrasound using blue protocol* to detect these changes in the form of more than normal number of B lines is prudent. If the patient is hemodynamically stable, obtaining a *high-resolution computed tomography (HRCT) of the lung* can reveal the interstitial edema or fibrosis more accurately. All these measures can be used as a caution to limit the dose and time of high concentration of delivered oxygen to avoid potential toxicity. Eye examination

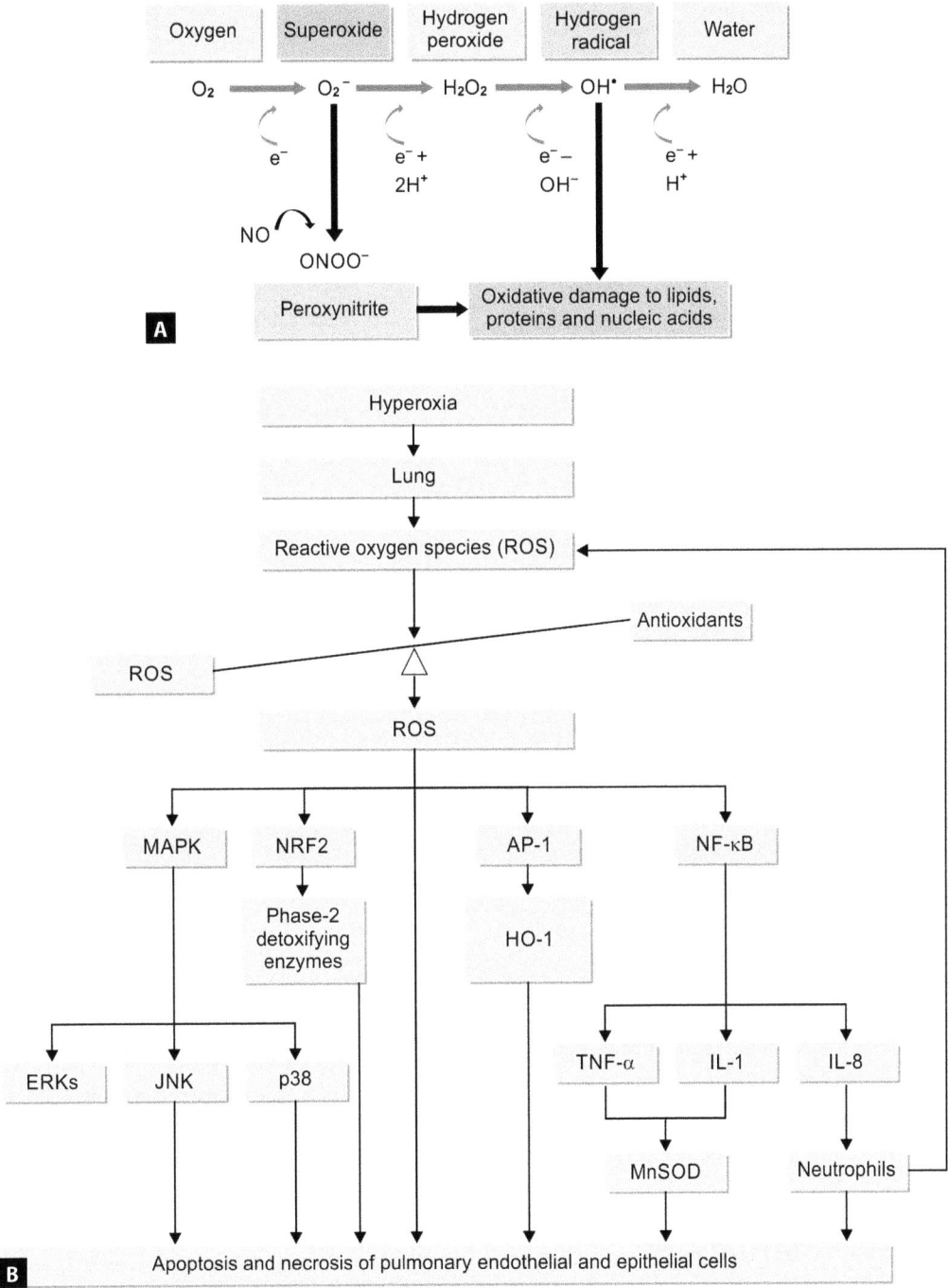

Figs. 1A and B: (A) Reduction of oxygen into reactive oxygen species, causing different effects on the lung tissue; (B) Pathophysiology of oxygen toxicity. (AP-1: activator protein 1; ERKs: extracellular signal-regulated kinases; HO-1: heme oxygenase-1; IL-1: interleukin-1; IL-8: interleukin 8; JNK: c-Jun N-terminal kinases; MAPK: mitogen-activated protein kinase; MnSOD: manganese superoxide dismutase; NF-κB: nuclear factor kappa B)

TABLE 1: Signs and symptoms of oxygen toxicity.

	Signs and Symptoms	
Central nervous system	**Pulmonary toxicity**	**Eyes**
Headache	Tracheobronchitis (exposure for >10 hour)	In neonates and premature babies (30-weeks' gestation or BW of 1,500 g), retinopathy of prematurity, retrolental fibroplasias, and intraventricular hemorrhages (FiO_2 >60%)
Altered behavior	Hemoptysis	Retinal edema
Hyperventilation (cogwheel breathing due to diaphragmatic twitching)	Dyspnea	Cataract formation (long-term exposure)
Hiccups, Cold shivering, facial pallor	Crepitations	Reversible progressive myopia
Fatigue	Fever	
Tingling in the limbs	Hyperemia of the nasal mucosa	
Visual changes—blurring and tunnel vision	Atelectasis	
Tinnitus and hearing disturbances	Diffuse alveolar hemorrhage	
Nausea		
Twitching of the perioral and small muscles of the hand (constant and early feature)		
Tonic–clonic seizure		
Amnesia		

(BW: birth weight; FiO_2: fraction of inspired oxygen)

for acuity and lens opacification forms an important pointer toward potential oxygen toxicity. A point to be noted here is that an electroencephalogram (EEG) is of no use in monitoring CNS symptoms.

PRESENT EVIDENCE AND SPECIFIC SITUATIONS

In hospitals, mortality was high in liberal oxygen therapy as compared to conservative in the meta-analysis of randomized controlled trials (RCTs) by Chu et al.

Myocardial Infarction

It is a well-known fact that ischemia reperfusion injury is caused due to the hyperoxia-induced coronary vasoconstriction and ROS.

Russek et al. in 1950 showed that the worsening of electrocardiogram (ECG) changes the suggestive of myocardial ischemia. Thomas et al. showed a correlation of decreased cardiac output with an increase in oxygen concentration. In a study by Sukumalchandra et al., it is revealed that oxygen transport and cardiac output do not improve in patients whose oxygen saturation is >90%. Routine administration of oxygen is not beneficial in the patients of nonhypoxic myocardial infarction (MI), as shown in a study by Rawles and group.

A study by Dion Stub et al. showed harmful effects of oxygen in ST-elevation myocardial infarction (STEMI) patients.

Hence, there are adequate signals to avoid routine administration of oxygen to patients with MI who are not hypoxic.

Post-Cardiac Arrest Scenario

Post-cardiac arrest syndrome (PCAS) develops in patients who are revived from the arrest situation. It behaves like multi-organ failure. Ischemia reperfusion injury and underlying disease state are responsible for PCAS. Excessive supplementation in a post-cardiac arrest situation can worsen the outcome due to release of ROS and hyperoxia-induced seizures. A study by Kilgannon et al. revealed that the hyperoxia group had a higher mortality than normoxia and hypoxia groups. Similar results were also shown in study by Bellomo et al. He defined hyperoxia as PaO_2 >300 mm Hg and hypoxia as PaO_2 <60 mm Hg. *Clinical practice guidelines recommend to maintain SpO_2 >94% in the post-cardiac arrest period.*

Stroke

There is no statistically significant difference between patients who receive oxygen and those who are not supplemented with oxygen.

TREATMENT

Management of the condition is purely symptomatic but remember that abrupt stoppage of oxygen at the onset of toxicity may aggravate the symptoms, which is also called the "oxygen off effect".

In ICU patients who are on a mechanical ventilator, try and get down with the FiO_2 to 60% or less as early as possible with target PaO_2 of 60 mm Hg and SpO_2 of even 90% to avoid deleterious effects of oxygen as described before. There has been some role of administering exogenous antioxidants, especially vitamins E and C. Also, a dietary supplement of trace elements such as selenium, zinc, and magnesium has been tried but it has not been of any use. For hyperbaric oxygen treatments, those at high risk may benefit from antiepileptic therapy, prolonged air breaks, and limited treatment pressure.

DIFFERENTIAL DIAGNOSIS

- CO_2 narcosis
- Carbon monoxide poisoning
- Toxin ingestion
- Cerebrovascular event
- Migraine
- Seizure disorder
- Infection
- Multiple sclerosis
- Hypoglycemia

PROGNOSIS

Removal of the inciting agent does not cause long-term neurological damage. Damage due to oxygen-induced pulmonary toxicity is reversible in most adults observed in long-term follow-up. Bronchopulmonary dysplasia in infants who survive will recover completely since the lungs continue to grow in the first 5–7 years, but are vulnerable for frequent respiratory infections in the future. Retinopathy is usually seen in premature infants and reverses without intervention in normal eyesight. In advanced cases, surgery intervention also has good results.

SUGGESTED READING

1. Callaway CW, Donnino MW, Fink EL, Golan E, Kern KB, Leary M, et al. Part 8: post cardiac arrest care: 2015 American Heart Association

Guidelines Update for Cardiopulmonary Resuscitation and Emergency Cardiovascular care. Circulation. 2015;132(18 Suppl 2):S465-82.
2. Chu DK, Kim LH, Young PJ, Zamiri N, Neary JD, Alhazzani W, et al. Mortality and morbidity in acutely ill adults treated with liberal versus conservative oxygen therapy (IOTA): a systematic review and meta-analysis. Lancet. 2018;391(10131):1693-705.
3. Ciencewicki J, Trivedi S, Kleeberger SR. Oxidants and the pathogenesis of lung diseases. J Allergy Clin Immunol. 2008;122(3):456-68.
4. Clanton TL. Hypoxia-induced reactive oxygen species formation in skeletal muscle. J Appl Physiol (1985). 2007;102(6):2379-88.
5. Davis WB, Rennard SI, Bitterman PB, Crystal RG. Pulmonary oxygen toxicity. Early reversible changes in human alveolar structures induced by hyperoxia. N Engl J Med. 1983;309(15):878-83.
6. Deneke SM, Fanburg BL. Normobaric oxygen toxicity of the lung. N Engl J Med. 1980;303(2):76-86.
7. Domachevsky L, Rachmany L, Barak Y, Rubovitch V, Abramovich A, Pick CG. Hyperbaric oxygen-induced seizures cause a transient decrement in cognitive function. Neuroscience. 2013;247:328-34.
8. Hafner S, Beloncle F, Koch A, Radermacher P, Asfar P. Hyperoxia in intensive care, emergency, and peri-operative medicine: Dr Jekyll or Mr Hyde? A 2015 update. Ann Intensive Care. 2015;5(1):42.
9. Mantell LL, Horowitz S, Davis JM, Kazzaz JA. Hyperoxia induced lung injury: correlation of apoptosis, necrosis, and inflammation. Ann N Y Acad Sci. 1999;887:171-80.
10. Martino GD, Luchetti M, De Rosa RC, Marroni A, Oriani G, Longoni C. Toxic effects of oxygen. In: Michael M, Marroni A. Longoni C (Eds). Handbook of Hyperbaric Medicine. New York: Springer; 1996. pp. 59-68.
11. Polderman KH. Mechanisms of action, physiological effects, and complications of hypothermia. Crit Care Med. 2009;37:S186-202.
12. Rahman I, Biswas SK, Kode A. Oxidant and antioxidant balance in the airways and airway diseases. Eur J Pharmacol. 2006;533(1-3):222-39.
13. Yee M, Vitiello PF, Roper JM, Staversky RJ, Wright TW, Finkelstein JN, et al. Type II epithelial cells are critical target for hyperoxia-mediated impairment of postnatal lung development. Am J Physiol Lung Cell Mol Physiol. 2006;291(5):L1101-11.

SECTION 4: Oxygen Targets

- **Effects of Hypoxia and Hypoxemia**
  Supradip Ghosh, Sonali Ghosh

- **How does Oxygen Therapy Work?**
  Deepak Govil, Divya Pal

- **Oxygen Therapy and Targets in Disease Specifics**
  Sachin Gupta, Deeksha Singh Tomar

Effects of Hypoxia and Hypoxemia

CHAPTER 21

Supradip Ghosh, Sonali Ghosh

INTRODUCTION

Hypoxia refers to a clinical condition in which tissues are unable to undergo aerobic metabolism, either due to lack of oxygen delivery or due to failure of oxygen-utilization mitochondrial level. Like all living organisms, in human beings too, physiological systems have evolved to ensure optimal delivery of oxygen to all cells. These include maintenance of arterial oxygen tension in the blood through adequate uptake of oxygen at pulmonary alveoli, maintenance of adequate hemoglobin concentration for carrying oxygen in the blood and adequate cardiac output, and blood flow to ensure that the oxygen carried by hemoglobin reaches tissues. Oxygen is utilized by the mitochondria, organelles present within cells ("aerobic metabolism").

Both increased oxygen level ("hyperoxia") and lack of it ("hypoxia") can be sensed by different chemoreceptors in the body, in turn producing necessary adjustments in the cardiovascular dynamics and ventilatory rates, thus ensuring appropriate tissue-oxygen supply. In addition, all nucleated cells respond to reduced oxygen availability by making necessary adjustments at the cellular level through the activation of preexisting proteins (within minutes of hypoxic episode) and by making systemic adjustments through regulation of gene transcription (within hours to days). In this chapter, we are going to discuss the effects of hypoxia on cells and the body's adaptive response to hypoxia.

HYPOXIA: MECHANISMS

One or more of the following mechanisms can produce tissue hypoxia:

- *Hypoxemic hypoxia:* Hypoxemia is defined as low partial pressure of oxygen (PaO_2) in the blood. The relationship between PaO_2 and arterial oxygen saturation of hemoglobin (SaO_2) is sigmoid-shaped. Thus, when PaO_2 falls below 60 mm Hg, there is a steep fall in the hemoglobin saturation, reducing the overall oxygen-carrying capacity of the blood. At the tissue level, this sigmoid shape of the oxyhemoglobin dissociation curve ensures maximum delivery of the available oxygen to the cells. Different mechanisms of hypoxemia are low PaO_2 in the atmosphere (e.g., at the summit of Mount Everest), hypoventilation, diffusion limitation through alveolar membrane, shunt or ventilation–perfusion mismatch.
- *Anemic hypoxia:* PaO_2 is normal but oxygen-carrying capacity is reduced because of low hemoglobin concentration.
- *Stagnant hypoxia:* PaO_2 and hemoglobin concentration are normal, but oxygen delivery to tissues is reduced because of circulatory dysfunction. Examples include

circulatory shock and impaired regional perfusion due to arterial occlusion.
- *Cytotoxic hypoxia:* It refers to the failure of mitochondria to utilize oxygen effectively despite adequate tissue oxygen delivery. Examples include late stages of sepsis and cyanide toxicity.

EFFECTS OF HYPOXIA ON CELLS

Lack of aerobic metabolism leads to a decreased generation of adenosine triphosphate (ATP) in the cells. Maintenance of homeostatic functions of the cells is dependent on adequate supply of ATP through the ATP-dependent ion channels such as Na^+/K^+-ATPase pump. In fact, maintenance of ion-pump functions consumes 20–80% of the cell's metabolic expenditure. Cell death occurs when production of ATP fails to meet energy demands of these ion pumps.

Impaired function of the Na^+/K^+-ATPase pump leads to increased intracellular $[Na^+]$, which in turn is exchanged with $[Ca^{2+}]$ **(Fig. 1)**. Uncontrolled $[Ca^{2+}]$ influx through voltage-gated $[Ca^{2+}]$ channels activates calcium-dependent phospholipases and proteases, leading to uncontrolled cell swelling, hydrolysis of different cellular components, and eventually to cell necrosis. Cells having increased ion-pump activities (e.g., neuronal cells) are more susceptible to hypoxic damage than others.

ADAPTATION TO HYPOXIA

When the availability of oxygen is compromised, several chemosensory mechanisms are activated in concert. These compensatory mechanisms include: (1) increased ventilation, (2) increased cardiac output, (3) switch from aerobic to anaerobic metabolism at cellular level, (4) promotion of increased vascularization, and (5) enhancement of the oxygen-carrying capacity by increasing hemoglobin concentration. Some of these adaptations are rapid; others may take many hours to several days.

Effects on Vascular Smooth Muscle

Peripheral vessels in the systemic circulation dilate in response to hypoxia. This improves oxygen delivery to the tissues by reducing resistance to blood flow. This effect is particularly evident in coronary and cerebral circulation. Moreover, peripheral vasodilatation improves venous return to the heart and can improve cardiac output.

In contrast, pulmonary vessels constrict in response to hypoxemia and shunt blood away from the poorly ventilated alveoli. This effect improves the ventilation–perfusion matching.

Carotid and Neuroepithelial Bodies

Afferent neurons in carotid bodies (present at the bifurcation of common carotid arteries) and neuroepithelial bodies (present at the bifurcation of bronchi) sense decreased supply of oxygen in the blood and environments, respectively. Through their efferent chemosensory fibers, they produce cardiorespiratory adjustments in response to low oxygen, thus increasing ventilation and cardiac output.

Adaptation at Cellular Level

At the cellular level, adaptation to hypoxia is brought about by two simultaneous processes—switching over to anaerobic metabolism to maintain supply of ATP and decreasing energy-consuming anabolic processes. Within minutes of hypoxia, cells respond by an increase in glycolytic activity through allosteric regulation of phosphofructokinase activity. In cases of chronic hypoxia, there is also overexpression of many glycolytic enzymes through hypoxia-inducible factor-1 (HIF-1)

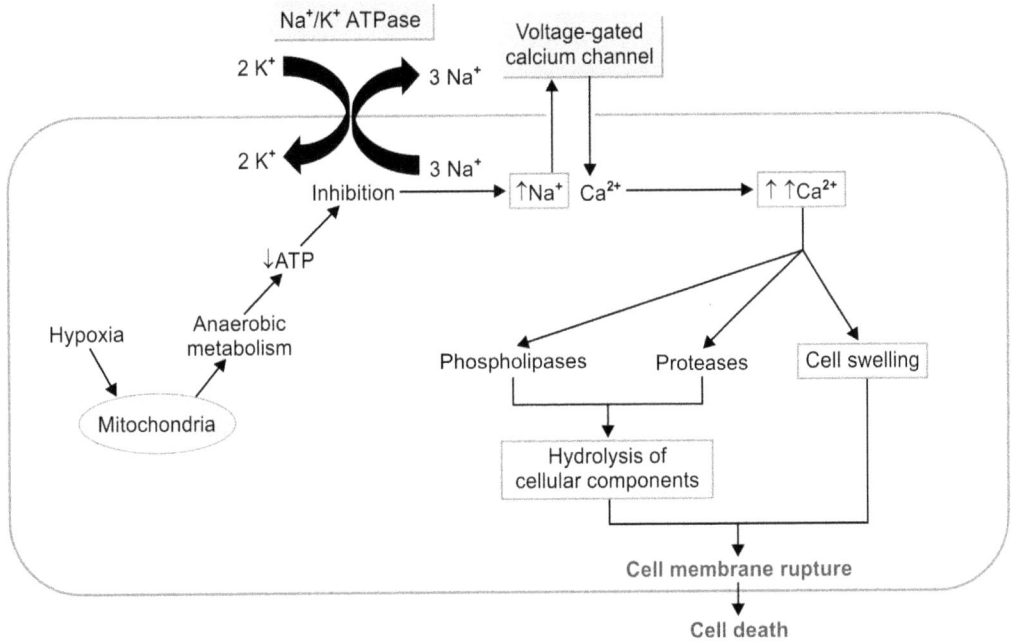

Fig. 1: Mechanisms of hypoxia-induced cell death. (ATP: adenosine triphosphate)

dependent pathway (explained later). Despite being less efficient (compared to oxidative phosphorylation in the mitochondria) in the generation of ATP, glycolysis can sustain cellular ionic activities in the presence of adequate supply of glucose. Protein synthesis and RNA/DNA synthesis are largely inhibited in the presence of hypoxia, as preserving Na^+/K^+-ATPase pump activity takes the priority. Mitochondrial respiratory chain function is inhibited in the presence of hypoxia.

AMP-kinase (AMPK) is the primary sensor in this cellular switching over function in response to hypoxia. Activation of AMPK stimulates translocation of glucose transporter type 4 (Glut-4) to plasma membrane, promoting increased cellular glucose uptake. In longer term, increased activity of AMPK also increases expression of Glut-4, hexokinase, and mitochondrial enzymes involved in the tricarboxylic acid cycle and respiratory chain. On the other hand, AMPK directly inhibits fatty acid, triglyceride and sterol synthesis and the expression of enzymes of fatty acid synthesis and gluconeogenesis.

Regulation of Gene Expression

Expression of several genes is upregulated in the presence of chronic hypoxia as a long-term adaptive mechanism. This includes (but not limited to) the following:

- *Tyrosine hydroxylase:* Involved in dopamine synthesis in carotid body cells
- *Glycolytic enzymes:* Phosphoglycerate kinase-1, pyruvate kinase, phosphofructokinase, aldolase A, glyceraldehyde 3-phosphate dehydrogenase, etc.
- *Glucose transporters:* Glut-1, Glut-4
- *Angiogenesis inducers:* Vascular endothelial growth factor (VEGF), platelet-derived growth factor (PDGF)
- *Nitric oxide synthase:* Increases vasodilation
- *Erythropoietin*: Increased production of RBCs

This transcriptional response is largely mediated by the activities of HIF-1. HIF-1 is a protein which is synthesized both in normoxic and in hypoxic conditions. However, it is degraded rapidly in the presence of normoxia but gets accumulated in the presence of hypoxia.

CLINICAL RELEVANCE

Cerebral Hypoxia

Brain is one of the most metabolically active organs, responsible for approximately 20% oxygen utilization (brain constitutes ~2% of body weight). Prolonged hypoxia leads to brain cell death, as a result of both necrosis and delayed apoptosis. In addition to mechanisms described above, influx of intracellular Ca^{2+} is enhanced further in the postsynaptic cells, due to the massive glutamate release from presynaptic neurons, in response to hypoxia.

In case of less severe hypoxia, neuronal cells can sustain for a longer duration by suppressing synthetic functions and spontaneous electrical activity ("penumbra"), provided oxygen supply is restored timely. Irreversible neuronal damage occurs if the hypoxia continues for more than 3 minutes. Susceptibility to hypoxic injury is substantially more in motor neurons compared to others. Unfortunately, reperfusion itself can induce neuronal death through generation of reactive oxygen species ("reperfusion injury").

Myocardial Ischemia

Myocardial cells also respond in a similar manner to hypoxia with prolonged hypoxia causing cell death. But unlike neuronal cells, they can sustain hypoxia for somewhat longer duration (up to 20 minutes).

Coronary reperfusion produces an interesting phenomenon in myocardial tissue called "myocardial stunning," which is characterized by prolonged postischemic dysfunction of reperfused tissue. Stunned myocardium is otherwise viable.

Optimal Oxygenation Target

Observational studies have shown a U-shaped relationship between PaO_2 values and ICU mortality, with both higher and lower PaO_2 values independently associated with increased mortality. Several randomized controlled trials have looked into the optimal oxygenation target in ICU patients with some showing benefits of conservative strategy ("Oxygen-ICU" trial) and others showing harm associated with it ["$LOCO_2$" (Liberal Oxygenation versus Conservative Oxygenation in Acute Respiratory Distress Syndrome) trial]. Some larger trials have shown overall equivocal results with benefits of conservative or liberal strategies in specific subgroup of patients ["ICU-ROX" (Intensive Care Unit Randomized Trial Comparing Two Approaches to Oxygen Therapy) trial, "HOT-ICU" (Handling Oxygenation Targets in the ICU) trial]. In a recent article, Young and colleagues have suggested the following recommendations based on current evidence:

- Both $PaO_2 < 60$ mm Hg and $PaO_2 > 110$ mm Hg should be avoided.
- Maintaining PaO_2 80–110 mm Hg is overall safe and may be preferred in patients with sepsis and in circulatory shock.
- Overall, PaO_2 target 60–80 mm Hg is safe and may be preferred in patients with hypoxic ischemic encephalopathy.

Tumor Angiogenesis

To sustain rapid growth, tumors must ensure adequate supply of oxygen to the rapidly growing tumor cells by growing new blood vessels ("neoangiogenesis"). This process is also important for the dissemination of tumor cells to distant sites ("metastasis"). Hypoxia present in the core of a tumor stimulates the accumulation of HIF-1. Moreover, HIF-1 is upregulated in a wide range of cancers. HIF-1, in turn, promotes angiogenesis through the expression of several angiogenic proteins with VEGF being the most potent one. In addition to promoting angiogenic proteins, HIF-1 also plays an important role in adaptation of tumor cells to hypoxia, as described above. Inhibition of HIF-1 can be a potential target for cancer therapy. Several HIF-1 inhibitors are in various stages of development for this purpose.

CONCLUSION

Persistent hypoxia beyond a few minutes causes irreversible damage to tissues, including cell death. However, human body has developed a robust system to sustain in the presence of mild hypoxia by making cardiovascular and respiratory adjustments, metabolic changes at the cellular level, and upregulation of certain genetic signals.

Deleterious effects of hyperoxia are also known, especially if it is sustained for a substantially long period, making it important for the clinician to choose a reasonable oxygenation target while prescribing oxygen therapy.

SUGGESTED READING

1. Young PJ, Hodgson CL, Rasmussen BS. Oxygen targets. Intensive Care Med. 2022;48(6):732-5.

How does Oxygen Therapy Work?

CHAPTER 22

Deepak Govil, Divya Pal

INTRODUCTION

Oxygen therapy is defined as administration of supplemental oxygen above that of atmospheric air with the aim to prevent and treat symptoms related to hypoxia. The ambient air at the sea level contains 21% oxygen, which decreases as the altitude increases. Oxygen is a drug—one of the most commonly used ones—which, like other drugs, has specific indications, pharmacokinetics, pharmacodynamics, spectrum of effective dosages, and side effects.

GOALS OF OXYGEN THERAPY

The objective of providing supplemental oxygen is to treat and prevent hypoxemia, thus taking care of the negative consequences of tissue hypoxia. Hypoxia can still be there even when hypoxemia has been taken care of, where sufficient amount of oxygen is not available at the tissue level to maintain homeostasis, for example in histotoxic hypoxia.

Hypoxia can result in potential irreversible organ damage, thus the importance of providing oxygen therapy. But, simultaneously, it is imperative to prevent hyperoxia and oxygen toxicity. Hypoxia may be associated with increased work of breathing and can also lead to pulmonary vasoconstriction, thus causing pulmonary hypertension. It can also result in myocardial ischemia, arrhythmias, hypotension, and lactic acidosis. The neurological effects of hypoxia, depending on its severity, include confusion, delirium, agitation, and coma.

HOW DOES OXYGEN THERAPY WORK?

In order to understand how supplemental oxygen can improve hypoxemia and the related insult, it is important to understand the oxygen transport and its delivery in physiology and in pathology.

Oxygen Transport and Delivery

Gas transfer across any membrane usually depends on the principle of diffusion, described as Fick's law of diffusion: oxygen diffusion = $K \times A/T \times \Delta P$, where A is the surface area of the membrane, T is the thickness, and ΔP is the partial pressure difference across the membrane. But because of poor solubility of oxygen in water (solubility of 0.003082 g/100 g H_2O), other methods (described as follows) also contribute to its delivery to tissues.

- Ventilation from the atmosphere to the lungs (alveoli) by convection:

    $$PAO_2 = FiO_2 \times (P_{atm} - PH_2O) - PaCO_2 / R,$$

    where PAO_2 is the partial pressure of oxygen in the ideal alveolus; FiO_2 is the fraction of oxygen in inspired gas; P_{atm} is the atmospheric pressure; PH_2O is saturated vapor pressure of water (47 mm Hg); $PaCO_2$ is the partial pressure of CO_2 in arterial blood; and R is the respiratory quotient (usually, 0.8). At the sea level, P_{atm} is 160 mm Hg and PAO_2 is 100 mm Hg.

CHAPTER 22: How does Oxygen Therapy Work?

Clinical pearls: Most of the times, the basis of oxygen therapy in either spontaneous or mechanical lung ventilation is increment in FiO_2. Exception to this can be seen in apneic oxygenation performed during anesthesia induction or apnea test for diagnosis of brain death, wherein bulk flow transfer of oxygen into the alveoli happens due to creation of oxygen-pressure gradient.

- From alveoli to blood—by diffusion across the alveolar-capillary membrane.
In health, PaO_2 (partial pressure of oxygen in pulmonary capillaries) approximates 90 mm Hg.

Clinical pearls: A-a gradient (PAO_2–PaO_2) depends on the effective membrane thickness and the surface area available for exchange, which is altered in critically ill patients (diffusion defect) and on the correlation between ventilation (V) and perfusion (Q) at the level of alveoli (V/Q mismatch). Right-to-left shunt and increasing age are associated with an increased A-a gradient.

- Saturation of hemoglobin (Hb) with oxygen (SaO_2) after diffusing into blood.
The SaO_2:PaO_2 relationship is sigmoidal in shape and the PaO_2 at which 50% of Hb is saturated with oxygen is P50.

Clinical pearls: Hyperthermia, hypercarbia, acidemia and increased 2,3-diphosphoglycerate (2,3-DPG, a byproduct of glycolysis, binds Hb mainly in hypoxic tissues) shift the Hb-O_2 dissociation curve for any given PO_2 to the right and facilitate the release of O_2 from Hb. While the converse happens with hypothermia, alkalosis, decreased PCO_2 and 2,3-DPG, methemoglobinemia, and carbon monoxide exposure, thus decreasing the oxygen release at tissues.

Supplemental oxygen therapy is usually indicated when PaO_2 falls to less than 60 mm Hg or the SaO_2 is less than 88%.

- From blood to tissues by convection, driven by the cardiovascular system (CVS) that is cardiac output (CO) centrally and regional tissue perfusion peripherally. The oxygen delivery (DO_2) also depends on its concentration in arterial blood (CaO_2).

$$DO_2 \text{ (mL/min)} = 10 \times CO \text{ (L/min)} \times CaO_2;$$
$$CaO_2 = [Hb \text{ (g/dL)} \times 1.39 \times SaO_2 \text{ (\%)}] + (0.003 \times PaO_2)$$

Oxygen consumption (VO_2) mL/min = 10 × CO (L/min) × (CaO_2–CvO_2) where CvO_2 is oxygen concentration in venous blood. Oxygen extraction ratio (OER): OER = VO_2/DO_2.

In health, at rest, DO_2 is 1,000 mL/min, VO_2 is 250 mL/min, and OER is 25%. At critical DO_2 (cDO_2), maximum OER is achieved, around 70%.

Clinical pearls: OER varies for different organs. Any increase in VO_2 or decrease in DO_2 beyond cDO_2 leads to tissue hypoxia, anaerobic metabolism, and increased lactate levels.

Increase in OER is indicative of decreased DO_2 (e.g., in hypoxic hypoxia, anemia, depressed cardiac function, shock, or hypoperfused state) or increased VO_2. (e.g., in inflammatory state such as sepsis, trauma, and burns; hypermetabolic state such as hyperthyroidism; increased muscular activity as in convulsions, exercise, shivering; and therapeutic interventions like adrenergic drugs.) Conversely, decreased OER is indicative of increased DO_2 (as in hyperoxic states—hyperbaric oxygen/high FiO_2) or decreased VO_2 (e.g., in histotoxic hypoxia, hypothyroidism, and sedation-paralysis).

The saturation of pulmonary artery, mixed venous blood (SvO$_2$ 70%), or central venous blood (ScvO$_2$ 68-77%) can be used as an indicator of adequate resuscitation of a critically ill patient and adequate DO$_2$. However, the possibility of a normal SvO$_2$ being suggestive of inadequate oxygen utilization (due to microcirculatory dysfunction as in cyanide poisoning or altered cellular oxygen uptake) rather than adequate oxygen delivery should be kept in mind.

- Blood to mitochondria—by diffusion.

Adenosine triphosphate (ATP) is generated by oxygen from the citric acid cycle. With decreased oxygen, there is anaerobic glycolysis and reduced ATP production.

Different Types of Hypoxia and Response to Oxygen Therapy

Based on the physiology of gas transport, we can now understand how oxygen therapy can or cannot help in different types of hypoxia.

- *Hypoxemic hypoxia:* Different mechanisms leading to hypoxemic hypoxia have been summarized in **Table 1**. Increasing FiO$_2$ can improve hypoxemia, except in the case of pulmonary shunt.
- *Anemic hypoxia:* Decrease in oxygen-carrying capacity of blood leads to this, implying that lesser Hb molecules or oxygen-binding sites are available to carry oxygen (as understood from the CaO$_2$ equation). Examples include anemia, decreased hematocrit, methemoglobinemia, and carbon monoxide poisoning. Since all the available oxygen-binding sites are fully saturated and PaO$_2$ is normal, respiratory chemoreceptors do not sense this defect and thus supplemental oxygen will not help in improving hypoxia, except in carbon monoxide poisoning where supplementing high FiO$_2$

TABLE 1: Role of oxygen therapy in hypoxic hypoxia.

Mechanism	PAO$_2$–PaO$_2$ gradient	PaCO$_2$	Response to oxygen therapy	Conditions associated
V/Q mismatch	Elevated	Variable	Good	Asthma, COPD, Pulmonary hypertension, interstitial lung disease (ILD)
Pulmonary shunt	Elevated	Normal	Poor	Pneumonia, pulmonary edema, acute respiratory distress syndrome (ARDS), alveolar collapse, and pulmonary arteriovenous communication
Diffusion limitation	Elevated	Usually Normal	Good	Emphysema, parenchymal lung disease
Hypoventilation	Normal	High	Good	Neuromuscular disorders: Impaired central drive/spinal cord level/nerve involvement supplying respiratory muscles (GBS), neuromuscular junction disease (MG, LES), myopathy, chest wall deformities
Low ambient oxygen	Normal	Reduced	Good	High altitude

(COPD: chronic obstructive pulmonary disease; GBS: Guillain–Barré syndrome; LES: Lambert–Eaton syndrome; MG: myasthenia gravis; PaCO$_2$: partial pressure of carbon dioxide; PAO$_2$: alveolar oxygen tension)

at atmospheric pressure or hyperbaric chamber can displace carbon monoxide from Hb.
- *Stagnant hypoxia:* Has its origin in CVS and occurs due to low blood flow, which can be local (ischemic perfusion) or global/systemic (decreased CO), leading to decreased DO_2. Supplemental oxygen does not reverse the hypoxia as PaO_2 is normal.
- *Histotoxic hypoxia:* Defect in cellular oxygen consumption leads to decrease in ATP generation by mitochondria despite adequate oxygen delivery, for example in cyanide poisoning. Decreased OER leads to increased SvO_2. Supplemental oxygen therapy does not reverse hypoxia.

Oxygen Therapy Devices

In spontaneously breathing hypoxic patients, oxygen delivery to alveoli is achieved by increasing FiO_2 using different variable- and fixed-performance devices available **(Table 2)**. FiO_2 delivered depends on certain patient factors [peak inspiratory flow rate (PIFR), presence/absence of respiratory pause, tidal volume generation] and certain device factors (oxygen flow rate, mask capacity, air vent size, interface fit). In critically ill hypoxic patients, increase in PIFR above 200 L/min and absence of respiratory pause can be seen, leading to decrease in alveolar FiO_2. This phenomenon is usual with variable performance masks but also seen with Venturi-type masks or

TABLE 2: Oxygen-delivery devices.

Low-flow systems	Variable performance	• Nasal cannula • Nasal catheter • Transtracheal catheter	• With flow 1 to 6 L/min, can deliver FiO_2 24–44%. • Keep flow <6 L/min; humidify if >4 L/min Difficult insertion • With flow 1/4 to 4 L/min, can provide FiO_2 22–35% • But needs surgical placement and is costly
Reservoir systems	Variable performance (Reservoir volume should be > the patient's tidal volume to provide fixed FiO_2)	• Reservoir cannula • Simple face mask • Partial rebreathing mask • Nonrebreathing mask • Tracheostomy mask	• Needs slightly less flow for target FiO_2 as compared to nasal cannula. Can provide FiO_2 24–45% • Can provide FiO_2 40–60% with flow of 5–8 L/min. Minimum flow 5 L/min required to avoid CO_2 rebreathing. Good for mouth breathers • Has no one-way valve between the reservoir bag and the mask. FiO_2 delivered ranges between 60–80%, needs gas flow >8 L/min. Bag to be kept inflated at all times to limit CO_2 rebreathing and ensure highest FiO_2. • Has unidirectional valves. Can deliver FiO_2 between 80–95% with gas flow between 10–15 L/min • Used in case of chronic oxygen therapy, provides good humidity
High-flow systems	Fixed performance	• Venturi mask • HFNC	• Can deliver FiO_2 between 24–60%, depending upon the jet orifice/connector selected. Particularly useful in patients with specific SpO_2 targets, e.g., COPD • The air-oxygen blender can allow FiO_2 delivery of up to 100%, with heated humidification available and flow can be generated up to 60 L/min.

(COPD: chronic obstructive pulmonary disease; FiO_2: fraction of inspired oxygen; HFNC: high-flow nasal cannula)

nonrebreather semirigid plastic masks with reservoir bags due to entrainment of room air. This can be overcome and a more predictable FiO_2 can be delivered by using high oxygen flow rates such as with high-flow nasal cannula (HFNC) or sealing the upper airway from the atmosphere [using continuous positive airway pressure (CPAP) or bilevel positive airway pressure (BiPAP) masks/ventilator] because they can match or exceed the patient's PIFR. So, patient's requirement and response to treatment should guide the use of nonsealing oxygen-delivery devices.

Targeted Oxygen Therapy

Oxygen therapy is an important part of initial resuscitation in critically ill patients, but proper identification of patients needing supplemental oxygen should be done and oxygen prescription should be individualized per patient **(Table 3)**.

TABLE 3: Oxygen therapy guidelines.

Conditions	Targeted oxygen therapy	Recommendations
Acute medical conditions except chronic hypercapnic states	Oxygen supplementation if SpO_2 <92% with target SpO_2 range 92–96% (grade C)	Thoracic Society of Australia and New Zealand (TSANZ) Guidelines, 2016
COPD and other chronic hypercapnic states	Oxygen supplementation if SpO_2 <88% with target SpO_2 range 88–92% (grade B)	Thoracic Society of Australia and New Zealand (TSANZ) Guidelines, 2016
Cardiac arrest	Use 100% Oxygen	ANZCOR
Bleomycin or paraquat toxicity	• Target of SpO_2 85% to reduce potentiation of lung injury by oxygen • The underlying causes of hypoxemia should be identified and treated. Oxygen should be given to treat hypoxemia, not dyspnea • Pulse oximetry shall be available in all clinical situations where oxygen is used for medical purposes and shall be used for regularly monitoring the supplemental oxygen therapy • The assessment of patients presenting with dyspnea shall include respiration rate, pulse rate, blood pressure, body temperature, mental state, as well as oxygen saturation. • Monitoring of oxygen by blood gas analyses should be performed in critically ill patients, ventilated patients, patients with severe hypoxemia, and risk of hypercapnia • Venous blood gas analysis shall not be used to monitor oxygen therapy. Venous blood gas analyses are able to exclude hypercapnia only at a $pvCO_2$ <45 mm Hg	• Thoracic Society of Australia and New Zealand (TSANZ) Guidelines, 2016 • German Guideline on Oxygen Therapy in Acute Care of Adults. Grade A • German Guideline on Oxygen Therapy in Acute Care of Adults. Grade A • German Guideline on Oxygen Therapy in Acute Care of Adults. Expert consensus • German Guideline on Oxygen Therapy in Acute Care of Adults. Expert consensus • German Guideline on Oxygen Therapy in Acute Care of Adults. Grade A

(ANZCOR: Australian and New Zealand Committee on Resuscitation; COPD: chronic obstructive pulmonary disease; $pvCO_2$: partial pressure of carbon dioxide in venous blood; SpO_2: oxygen saturation)

OXYGEN THERAPY HAZARDS

- *Related to supply:* Risk of explosion, combustion, and barotrauma (if administered directly at delivery pressures)
- Oxygen toxicity
- *Hyperoxia-induced vasoconstriction:* In cerebral, renal, coronary vasculature, and decreasing DO_2 to vital organs (except in pulmonary vasculature where hypoxia induces vasoconstriction)
- *Central nervous system (CNS) toxicity:* Acute neurological signs, seizures when exposed to oxygen delivered at high pressure (≈300 kPa), seen in diving
- *Pulmonary toxicity/injury:* Seen as decreased compliance, interstitial edema, and fibrosis (Lorraine–Smith Effect). Other pulmonary effects include V/Q mismatch, absorption atelectasis, and a possible decreased ventilatory drive in chronic obstructive pulmonary disease (COPD) patients.

CONCLUSION

Oxygen although essential for life, but when prescribed for therapy, it should be used carefully to improve hypoxia and simultaneously avoid hyperoxia. It is important to understand the physiological effects of oxygen supplementation and different oxygen delivery devices available.

SUGGESTED READING

1. Australian Resuscitation Council and New Zealand Resuscitation Council. (2016). ANZCOR guidelines. ANZCOR guideline 11.6.1—Targeted oxygen therapy in adult advanced life support. [online] Available from https://inmedes.com.ua/wp-content/uploads/2020/01/anzcor-guideline-11-6-1-targeted-oxygen-therapy-jan16.pdf [Last accessed June, 2022].
2. Beasly R, Chien J, Douglas J, Eastlake L, Farah C, King G, et al. Thoracic Society of Australia and New Zealand (TSANZ): Oxygen guidelines for acute oxygen use in adults. Respirology. 2015;20(8):1182-91.
3. Bitterman H. Bench-to-bedside review: oxygen as a drug. Crit Care. 2009;13(1):205.
4. Gottlieb J, Capetian P, Hamsen U, Janssens U, Karagiannidis C, Kluge S, et al. German S3 guideline: oxygen therapy in the acute care of adult patients. Respiration. 2022;101:214-52.
5. Hardavella G, Karampinis I, Frille A, Sreter K, Rousalova I. Oxygen devices and delivery systems. Breathe. 2019;15:e108-16.
6. Junn J-OC, Mythen MG, Grocott MP. Physiology of oxygen transport. BJA Educ. 2016;16(10):341-8.
7. O'Driscoll BR, Howard LS, Earis J, Mak V; British Thoracic Society Emergency Oxygen Guideline Group; BTS Emergency Oxygen Guideline Development Group. BTS guideline for oxygen use in adults in healthcare and emergency settings. Thorax. 2017;72(Suppl 1):ii1-90.
8. Sampson B, Bihari S. Oxygen therapy. In: Bersten A, Handy JM (Eds). Oh's Intensive Care Manual, 8th edition. Elsevier Limited; 2018.
9. Sarkar M, Niranjan N, Banyal PK. Mechanisms of hypoxemia. Lung India. 2017;34:47-60.

Oxygen Therapy and Targets in Disease Specifics

CHAPTER 23

Sachin Gupta, Deeksha Singh Tomar

INTRODUCTION

Oxygen is the most commonly prescribed drug to a patient and it seems most benign as far as side effects are concerned. Oxygen therapy is an important aspect in management of critically ill patients but this therapy also has its limits and targets. Both hyperoxia and hypoxemia have the potential to harm critically ill patients and also have an impact on their outcomes. The age old concept of "more is better" was being followed for oxygen therapy as there was no way to judge the optimum oxygen requirement of a patient unless an arterial blood gas was done. There have been many trials which have shown the high concentration of oxygen in the blood (hyperoxia) is associated with harmful effects and hence should be avoided.

Critical care units cater to various subset of patients and hence forming a universal oxygen therapy strategy may not seem justifiable. The targets of oxygen therapy are individualized as per the disease state **(Table 1)**.

DISEASE STATES

Myocardial Ischemia

The concept of increasing oxygen concentration in vascular occlusive state like myocardial ischemia (MI) seems logical as it will increase the oxygen concentration in the ischemic tissues, but hyperoxia leads to tissue damage by generation of reactive oxygen species.

TABLE 1: Oxygen targets for different disease states.

Disease states	Oxygen target
Myocardial ischemia	Oxygen supplementation if SpO_2 <90% in STEMI and NSTEMI
Traumatic brain injury	Oxygen supplementation to target SpO_2 >94%
Stroke	Oxygen supplementation to target SpO_2 >94%
Hypoxic ischemic encephalopathy	Oxygen supplementation to target SpO_2 >94%
COPD	Target SpO_2 88–92%
ARDS	Target SpO_2 >88%
ICU-ventilated patients	Restrictive oxygen administration to target SpO_2 >94% or PaO_2 >60 mm Hg
Sepsis	Optimum target of oxygen administration not certain

(ARDS: acute respiratory distress syndrome; COPD: chronic obstructive pulmonary disease; ICU: intensive care unit; NSTEMI: non-ST-segment elevation myocardial infarction; STEMI: ST-elevation myocardial infarction)

The AVOID (Air Verses Oxygen In myocardial infarction) trial conducted in patients with ST-segment elevation confirmed that normoxic patients who received supplemental oxygen had higher levels of cardiac enzymes and larger infarct size, higher reinfraction rate, and arrythmias as confirmed on magnetic resonance imaging.

The DETO2X-AMI (DETermination of the Role of Oxygen in Suspected Acute Myocardial Infarction) study was conducted in non-ST-segment elevation myocardial infarction (NSTEMI). The patients who were given oxygen only when oxygen saturation measured by pulse oximetry was <90% did not have an increase in mortality, rate of reinfarction, arrhythmias, or shock as compared to the oxygen group who received fixed 6 L/min oxygen.

The supplemental oxygen can lead to increase in coronary vascular resistance, reduced coronary blood flow, and more generation of reactive oxygen species leading to vasoconstriction and reperfusion injury. On the basis of these two trials, the European and American guidelines have recommended that oxygen supplementation should only be given when peripherally measured oxygen saturation is <90%.

Neurological Conditions

Traumatic Brain Injury

The major goal of management in neurointensive care is to avoid secondary brain injury. Correction of hypoxemia forms an important aspect of it. In patients with traumatic brain injury, the brain tissue oxygenation levels are lower and are associated with worse outcomes, hence the practice of liberal oxygen therapy may increase the brain tissue oxygenation levels. But the ICU-ROX (Intensive Care Unit Randomized Trial Comparing Two Approaches to Oxygen Therapy) trial which had a subgroup of acute brain pathologies failed to reveal any significant difference in 90-day mortality between the conservative and liberal groups.

Stroke

There have been few randomized trials which have evaluated at the role of oxygen therapy in ischemic stroke patients. The SO_2S study which enrolled 8,003 stroke patients concluded that there was no difference in modified Rankin Scale (mRS) scores between the groups which received oxygen and which did not.

Hypoxic Ischemic Encephalopathy

The secondary injury occurring after resuscitation postcardiac arrest is due to generation of oxygen free radical production. The liberal provision of oxygen may give rise to further oxygen radical production, cellular injury, apoptosis, and neuronal death. The animal models have shown worse neurological deficit in patients who have received 100% oxygen postresuscitation. The ICU-ROX trial concluded that 45% patients who received conservative oxygen had favorable outcome on the Extended Glasgow Outcome Scale at 180 days as compared to 32% who received liberal oxygen.

On the basis of evidence present, it is now recommended to keep oxygen saturation above 94% in patients with stroke and oxygen to be given only if above target not met.

Pulmonary Conditions

Chronic Obstructive Pulmonary Disease

The guidelines have recommended to target the peripherally measured oxygen saturation of 88–92% by pulse oximetry. The findings of randomized controlled trial (RCT) which compared liberal versus titrated oxygen therapy in patients with acute exacerbations of emphysema revealed that titrated oxygen therapy reduced mortality by 58% in all patients and 78% in patients with confirmed chronic obstructive pulmonary disease (COPD). Liberal oxygen administration is associated with increased incidence of respiratory acidosis and high-mortality probably due to worsening ventilation/

perfusion mismatch. Overzealous oxygen administration leads to reduction in ventilatory drive due to abolishment of hypoxic pulmonary vasoconstriction.

Acute Respiratory Distress Syndrome

Acute respiratory distress syndrome (ARDS) patients are hypoxemic and generally require oxygen as a part of their treatment regime. To achieve a safe minimum oxygen level in blood, these patients may still require liberal oxygen therapy, and may be prone to oxygen toxicity. The liberal oxygen protocol may give rise to supranormal oxygen levels and impair macrophage function. These mechanisms lead to increase in ventilation/perfusion mismatch.

The oxygen therapy in ARDS patients was compared in the Liberal Oxygenation versus Conservative Oxygenation in Acute Respiratory Distress Syndrome (LOCO$_2$) trial. This trial had to be stopped prematurely due to safety concerns as there were increased mortality (44 vs. 30.4%) at 90 days in the conservative group. Although there were many caveats in interpretation of this finding as the conservative group had 88% of saturation as the endpoint as compared to 96% in the liberal group. So such hypoxemic patients are more prone to worsening in episodes like suctioning or inadvertent ventilator disconnection. This is probably the only trial which enrolled ARDS patients.

The ICU-ROX trial was done on hypoxic respiratory failure patients with pulse oximetry/fraction of inspired oxygen (PF) ratio of <300 mm Hg. This study concluded that there was no difference in ventilator-free alive days between the conservative and the liberal group. The reason could be a very narrow difference between the oxygen targets of both the groups.

The largest trial, the Handling Oxygenation Targets in the ICU (HOT-ICU) trial, enrolled 2,928 patients with acute hypoxemic respiratory failure. The trial could not find any mortality difference (42.9 vs. 42.4%) at 90 days between lower oxygenation group (partial pressure of oxygen, PaO$_2$ of 60 mm Hg) versus the higher oxygenation group (PaO$_2$ of 90 mm Hg).

The target of oxygen therapy in ARDS and other hypoxemic states is still a matter of debate and has not reached any consensus. The available data suggests that down regulating the oxygen therapy in severe hypoxemic patients should not be followed and one should try achieving a saturation level of 88% and above within the best safest oxygen level provided to the patient.

GENERAL INTENSIVE CARE VENTILATED PATIENTS

The nonhypoxemic ventilated patients generally do not require high-oxygen support but still there has no strict recommendations on the optimum oxygen concentration in these patients. The OXYGEN-ICU trial compared the conservative oxygen therapy (PaO$_2$ between 70 and 100 mm Hg) versus the conventional care group (PaO$_2$ >150 mm Hg). The study concluded that the conservative therapy group had shorter intensive care unit (ICU) length of stay and lower mortality as compared to the other group (11.6 vs. 20%).

In another trial by Panwar et al., there was no difference in mortality or other organ dysfunction between the conservative strategy (SpO$_2$ 88–92%) group and the liberal strategy (SpO$_2$ >96%) group.

On the basis of these two trials, the practice is to follow the conservative strategy of oxygen therapy to achieve normoxia.

Sepsis

The oxygen consumption of the body increases during a septic insult. The fundamental of providing liberal oxygen to septic patient seems justifiable as the oxidative killing of bacteria is enhanced by the increased production of neutrophil superoxide in the presence of high oxygen concentration.

As per the ICU-ROX trial, there was 7% point nonsignificant decrease in mortality in the liberal strategy group in septic patients as compared to the conservative group. Although this data cannot guide us to give hyperoxia to septic patients. In the French trial, hyperoxia and hypertonic saline in patients with septic shock (HYPERS2S) trial, patients were randomized to receive mechanical ventilation with either fraction of inspired concentration of oxygen (FiO_2) at 1.0 (hyperoxia group) or the FiO_2 was set to target PaO_2 of 88–95% (normoxia group). The trial was stopped prematurely as the hyperoxia group showed higher mortality (43 vs. 35%), increased incidence of ICU-acquired weakness (11 vs. 6%), and increased atelectasis (12 vs. 6%). They concluded that arterial hyperoxia should not be induced in septic patients.

On the basis of these trials, further research is warranted to document the optimum concentration of oxygen required in septic patients. Still, it is clear that hyperoxia should be avoided as it has not shown any benefit in this specific subgroup.

OXYGEN THERAPY IN INTENSIVE CARE UNIT

There has been no clear-cut answers to the question that "what is the optimum level of oxygen that a patient should be given?" As per the Cochrane review by Barbateskovic et al., there has been no strong evidence to suggest that hyperoxia is associated with improved outcomes in critically ill patients. Rather, the trend is toward harm with increase in mortality. The ongoing Mega-ROX trial is intended to compare conservative and liberal strategies of oxygen therapy in mechanically ventilated patients.

CONCLUSION

There is enough evidence to suggest that misuse of oxygen therapy is done in most of the critical care units as the harmful effects of hyperoxia are not visible immediately. Although the disease state of the patient will guide the oxygen therapy but most of the evidence present suggest that maintaining normoxia in the patient should be the goal and this should be achieved at the lowest possible oxygen therapy. Bedside pulse oximetry should be used to assess the peripheral oxygen saturation if the arterial blood gas is not available or not feasible.

SUGGESTED READING

1. Amsterdam EA, Wenger NK, Brindis RG, Casey DE Jr, Ganiats TG, Holmes DR Jr, et al. 2014 AHA/ACC guideline for the management of patients with non-ST-elevation acute coronary syndromes: a report of the American College of Cardiology/American Heart Association Task Force on Practice Guidelines. Circulation. 2014;130:e344-426.
2. Asfar P, Schortgen F, Boisrame-Helms J, Charpentier J, Guerot E, Megarbane B, et al. Hyperoxia and hypertonic saline in patients with septic shock (HYPERS2S): a two-by-two factorial, multicentre, randomised, clinical trial. Lancet Respir Med. 2017;5(3): 180-90.
3. Austin MA, Wills KE, Blizzard L, Walters EH, Wood-Baker R. Effect of high flow oxygen on mortality in chronic obstructive pulmonary disease patients in prehospital setting: randomised controlled trial. BMJ. 2010;341:c5462.
4. Barbateskovic M, Schjørring OL, Russo Krauss S, Jakobsen JC, Meyhoff CS, Dahl RM, et al. Higher versus lower fraction of inspired oxygen or targets of arterial oxygenation for adults admitted to the intensive care unit. Cochrane Database Syst Rev. 2019;2019(11):CD012631.

5. Barrot L, Asfar P, Mauny F, Winiszewski H, Montini F, Badie J, et al. Liberal or conservative oxygen therapy for acute respiratory distress syndrome. N Engl J Med. 2020;382(11):999-1008.
6. Girardis M, Busani S, Damiani E, Donati A, Rinaldi L, Marudi A, et al. Effect of conservative vs. conventional oxygen therapy on mortality among patients in an intensive care unit: the Oxygen-ICU randomized clinical trial. JAMA. 2016;316:1583-9.
7. Hofmann R, James SK, Jernberg T, Lindahl B, Erlinge D, Witt N, et al. Oxygen therapy in suspected acute myocardial infarction. New Engl J Med. 2017;377:1240-9.
8. Ibanez B, James S, Agewall S, Antunes MJ, Bucciarelli-Ducci C, Bueno H, et al. 2017 ESC guidelines for the management of acute myocardial infarction in patients presenting with ST-segment elevation: the task force for the management of acute myocardial infarction in patients presenting with ST-segment elevation of the European Society of Cardiology (ESC). Eur Heart J. 2018;39(2):119-77.
9. Mackle D, Bellomo R, Bailey M, Beasley R, Deane A, Eastwood G, et al.; ICU-ROX Investigators the Australian and New Zealand Intensive Care Society Clinical Trials Group. Conservative oxygen therapy during mechanical ventilation in the ICU. N Engl J Med. 2020;382(11):989-98.
10. O'Driscoll BR, Howard LS, Earis J, Mak V. BTS guideline for oxygen use in adults in healthcare and emergency settings. Thorax. 2017;72(Suppl 1):ii1-ii90.
11. Panwar R, Hardie M, Bellomo R, Barrot L, Eastwood GM, Young PL, et al. Conservative versus liberal oxygenation targets for mechanically ventilated patients. A pilot multicenter randomized controlled trial. Am J Respir Crit Care Med. 2016;193(1):43-51.
12. Pilcher J, Weatherall M, Shirtcliffe P, Bellomo R, Young P, Beasley R. The effect of hyperoxia following cardiac arrest - a systematic review and meta-analysis of animal trials. Resuscitation. 2012;83(4):417-22.
13. Powers WJ, Rabinstein AA, Ackerson T, Adeoye OM, Bambakidis NC, Becker K, et al. Guidelines for the early management of patients with acute ischemic stroke: 2019 update to the 2018 guidelines for the early management of acute ischemic stroke: a guideline for healthcare professionals from the American Heart Association/American Stroke Association. Stroke. 2019;50(12):e344-e418.
14. Roffe C, Nevatte T, Crome P, Gray R, Sim J, Pountain S, et al. The Stroke Oxygen Study (SO_2S) - a multi-center, study to assess whether routine oxygen treatment in the first 72 hours after a stroke improves long-term outcome: study protocol for a randomized controlled trial. Trials. 2014;15:99.
15. Schjorring OL, Klitgaard TL, Perner A, Wetterslev J, Lange T, Siegemund M, et al. Lower or higher oxygenation targets for acute hypoxemic respiratory failure. N Engl J Med. 2021;384:1301-11.
16. Stub D, Smith K, Bernard S, Nehme Z, Stephenson M, Bray JE, et al.; AVOID Investigators. Air versus oxygen in ST-segment-elevation myocardial infarction. Circulation. 2015;131(24):2143-50.

Index

Page numbers followed by *b* refer to box, *f* refer to figure, *fc* refer to flowchart, and *t* refer to table.

A

Abscess, intracranial 112
Academia, workup of 86*fc*
Acetazolamide 86
Acid-base disorders 80, 81*t*
Acidemia 129
Acidosis 56, 80
Activator protein 117
Acute respiratory distress
 syndrome 28, 40, 81,
 134, 136
Adenosine triphosphate 51,
 124, 125
Adrenergic drugs 129
Aerobic metabolism 123
Air 10, 12, 18
 emboli 111
 entrainment, adjustment of 96
 separation unit 3, 6, 23, 30
Albumin correction 83
Alkalemia 85
 management of 87*fc*
Alkalosis 80
Alveolar gas equation 49
Alveolar hypoventilation 51, 71
Alveolar membrane 71
Alveolar septum 116
Alveolar-arterial gradient 49, 71
Alveolar-capillary membrane 129
Ambient light 78
Analeptics 84
Anemia 72, 78
 acute blood loss 111
Anemic anoxia 62
Anemic hypoxia 51, 123, 130
Anesthesia 28
Angiogenesis inducers 125
Anion gap 86
 concept of 84*f*
 high 86
Anoxic anoxia 61
Anxiety 84

Arterial blood gas 71, 80, 80*t*, 82
 analysis 80
Arterial carbon dioxide tension 61
Arterial insufficiency 112
Atelectasis 28
Avagadro's law 17

B

Barbeau test 76
Barometric otitis 113
Barotrauma 113
Beer-Lambart law 73
Bernoulli's principle 95
Bicarbonate 80
 conservation 83*f*
Bilevel positive airway pressure 41
Biphosphoglycerate 66
Bleomycin 132
Blood
 glucose 80
 oxygen content of 50
 plasma 64
 pressure, monitoring
  systolic 76
Bohr effect 60, 66
Boyle's law 110
Brain injury, traumatic 134, 135
Bubble humidifier 100
Burns 79

C

Capillary transit time 70
Carbon dioxide 10, 12, 18, 47, 55,
 57, 67, 69, 80, 93
Carbon dioxide dissociation
 curve 57*f*
Carbon dioxide retention 55-57
Carbon dioxide, pressure of 67
Carbon monoxide 67
Carbon monoxide antagonism 110
Carbon monoxide exposure 129

Carbon monoxide hemoglobin
 dissociation curve 67*f*
Carbon monoxide poisoning 28,
 51, 111
Carbonic acid 85
Carboxyhemoglobin 73, 110
Cardiopulmonary illness, acute 28
Catecholamine 84
Central nervous system 71,
 113, 133
Cerebral hypoxia 126
Cerebrospinal fluid 56
Chamber attendants, risk to 113
Chest trauma 28
Chloride responsive 87
Chloride unresponsive 87
Chronic obstructive pulmonary
 disease 30, 32, 52, 57, 81,
 105, 130, 131, 134, 135
Cilia, function of 99
Cirrhosis 81
Clostridium
 myonecrosis 111
 perfringens 111
Cold-water humidifier 100
Compartment syndromes 112
Compression injury 112
Conservative oxygen therapy 52
Continuous positive airway
 pressure 41
Convective oxygen transport 59
Corneal abrasions 79
Coronary vasoconstriction 52
COVID-19 40, 103
 pandemic 3, 16
Crush injury 112
Cryogenic air separation
 unit 3, 4*fc*
Cryogenic fractional distillation
 method 23*f*, 28
Cryogenic liquid 22
 cylinders 25
 medical oxygen 22

Index

Cyanide poisoning 51
Cyclopropane 12, 18
Cylinders
   components of 16
   connections 36
   handling of 36
   identification of 18
   testing of 17
   transportation of 36
Cytochrome oxidase 51
Cytopathic hypoxia 62
Cytotoxic hypoxia 124

D

Dead space ventilation 71
Decompression sickness 111
Deoxyhemoglobin 51, 73
Dephlogisticated air 22
Deployable oxygen concentration system 3, 5
Depression 71
Diabetic ketoacidosis 84
Diameter index safety system 11, 11f, 25, 26
Diarrhea 86
   severe 81
Diffusion capacity, measurement of 70
Diffusive oxygen transport 62
Diphosphoglycerate 60, 61, 66, 67
Disposable probes 75t
Domiciliary oxygen therapy 38
Dual lumen cannula barbs 26f
Duplex vacuum pump 14f
Dysrhythmias 77

E

Ear 113
Electrical interference 78
Endotracheal tube 99
Enterocutaneous fistulas 86
Entonox 12
Enzymes, function of 116
Erythropoietin 125
Ethylene 18
   glycol 84
External flow control valve 25

F

Face mask
   partial rebreather 93, 93f
   simple 93

Fetal hemoglobin 67
Fick's law 48, 62, 69
Fire hazard analysis, components of 37b
Fire triad 35f
Flickering lights 78
Flow control knob 26f
Fluid responsiveness 76

G

Gamma-amino butyric acid 116
Gas 8, 10, 12, 18
   bubble size reduction 110
   exchange, physiology of 47
   gangrene 111
Gene expression, regulation of 125
Glucose transporters 125
Glutamic acid 116
Glycolytic enzymes 125
Guillain-Barré syndrome 130

H

Haldane effect 58, 60
Hazard analysis 36
Headache 118
Hearing loss, idiopathic acute sensory 112
Heart failure, chronic 72
Heat and moisture exchanger filter 100
Helium 18
Hemodynamic therapy, goal-directed 63
Hemoglobin 59, 64, 88, 123
   capacity of 70
   low 51
   molecule 59f
   S 77
   saturation of 129
   structure of 59f
Henry's law 64, 110
High-flow nasal cannula 96, 97f, 101, 103, 107
   oxygen therapy 104f
High-flow nasal oxygen 101
High-flow systems 91fc, 131
Histotoxic hypoxia 51, 62, 129, 131
Hormones 84
Humidification 99, 105
   devices, types of 100
   physiology 99
   risks of 101
   system 100

Humidifiers, heated 100
Humidity 99
Hyperalimentation 86
Hyperbaric oxygen 129
   therapy 28, 109
      mechanism of action of 110
Hyperbaric therapy 109
Hyperbilirubinemia 78
Hypercapnia 56, 81
Hypercapnic respiratory failure 53, 105
Hypercarbia 129
Hyperchloremic metabolic acidosis 85
Hyperoxemia 76
Hyperoxia 123, 133
   effects of 127
Hyperoxic acute lung injury 116
Hyperoxic states 129
Hyperthermia 129
Hypotension 81
Hypothyroidism 129
Hypoventilation 49, 130
Hypovolemia 77
Hypoxemia 51, 56, 84, 128
   cause of 49
   effects of 123
   etiology of 49, 49t
Hypoxemic hypoxia 51, 123, 130
Hypoxia 123, 125, 128
   adaptation to 124
   effects of 123
   type of 61, 130
Hypoxic episode 123
Hypoxic hypoxia 130t
Hypoxic ischemic encephalopathy 134, 135
Hypoxic respiratory failure 105
Hypoxic tissues 129

I

Industrial oxygen 5
Inflammatory lung disease, chronic 96
Infrared interference 78
Inspired oxygen, fraction of 136
Intensive care unit 12, 40

K

Keratinization 99
Kidneys 83f
Krogh's cylinder model 62
Kyphoscoliosis 71

L

Lambert-Eaton syndrome 130
Liberal oxygen therapy 52
Liquid medical oxygen 24, 42
   tank 14, 24, 24f
Liquid oxygen 20, 23, 24, 30
   benefits of 28
   cryogenic production of 23f
   cylinders 28
   dewars 27
   limitations of 28
   plant 23
   storage tanks 28
Lung 55, 113
   primary function of 47

M

Mechanical ventilation 84
Medical air 14
   components of 14
Medical gas
   cylinders 16, 18t, 21
   pipeline system 8, 22
      components of 9f
Medical oxygen 5, 22, 40
Medical piped gas structure 8
Metabolic acidosis 83-85
   causes of
      hyperchloremic 85
      normal anion gap 85b
      high anion gap 85b
Metabolic alkalosis 87t
Metabolic disorders 80
Metaplasia 99
Metastasis 126
Methanol 84
Methemoglobin 73
Methemoglobinemia 129
Mitochondria 59
Monoplace chambers 109, 109f
Motion artifacts 78
Multiplace hyperbaric
      chamber 110f
Myasthenia gravis 130
Myocardial infarction 118
Myocardial ischemia 126, 134

N

Nail polish 78
Nasal cannula 92
Nasal catheter 92, 92f

Nasal low-flow oxygen,
      long-term 100
Nasal mucosa 99
Near-infrared spectroscopy 51
Necrotizing fasciitis 111
Neoangiogenesis 126
Neuroepithelial bodies 124
Neurointensive care,
      management in 135
Neuromuscular weakness 71
Neuronal cells 124
Nitric oxide synthase 125
Nitrogen 18, 110
Nitrous oxide 10, 12, 18
Nocturnal oxygen therapy trial 30
Noninvasive ventilation 100, 103
Nonrebreather mask 94, 94f, 106
Non-ST-segment elevation
      myocardial infarction
      134, 135
Nuclear magnetic resonance
      spectrometry 51

O

Obstructive sleep apnea 32
Optimal oxygenation target 126
Oxygen 3, 10, 12, 18, 22, 23, 35, 59,
   62, 64, 94, 134
   audit 40, 41
   basic facts of 1
   binding capacity 61
   carriers
      artificial 63
      hemoglobin based 63
   cascade 48f
   consumption 50, 62, 129
   content 50, 61
   diffuses 69
   diffusion of 69
   ecosystem 40
   enrichment, causes of 36b
   extraction ratio 62
   gas cylinders, sizes of 18t
   hazards of 35, 36t
   increased delivery of 110
   leaks 38
   manifold design 13
   overzealous 136
   partial pressure of 56
   pressure gradient 129
   production technologies 5, 6t
   regulator 37f
   requirement 40
   sources 29t

   species, reactive 116
   stewardship program 40, 41
   storage 37
   targets 53, 121, 134t
   transfer of 59
   utilization of 59, 91
Oxygen concentrator 3, 5, 5fc, 6,
   29, 30, 32, 33f, 34
   advantages of 34
   components of 32
   disadvantages of 34
   home users of 34
   types of 32, 33t
Oxygen cylinder 36
   filling 43
   storage of 36
Oxygen delivery 36, 37, 50, 61t
   devices 91, 131t
   equipment 22
   systems 12, 89
Oxygen therapy 35, 97, 99, 128,
   130, 134, 137
   cardinal goal of 51
   devices 131
   goals of 51, 52, 128
   guidelines 132t
   hazards 133
   humidification of 99
   long-term 28
   monitoring of 45
   physiology of 45
   role of 130t
   targeted 132
Oxygen toxicity 113, 115
   diagnosis 116
   differential diagnosis 119
   pathophysiology of 115, 117f
   prognosis 119
   severe cases of 115
   signs of 118t
   symptoms of 118t
   treatment 119
Oxygen transport 37, 59
   and delivery 128
Oxyhemoglobin 51, 73
   dissociation curve 60, 60f, 61t,
      64, 65, 65f, 66, 66f, 66t

P

Paraquat toxicity 132
Peripheral oxygen saturation 57
Peripheral pulses 80
Persistent hypoxia 127
Pin index system 11, 12, 17

Piped gas system, components of 8
Plasma membrane 125
Pneumonia 28
Pneumothorax 28
Portable fill connector 26f
Portable liquid oxygen dewar 25
Portable oxygen concentrator 30, 31, 33f
Positive end-expiratory pressure 96, 104
Post-cardiac arrest 119
Postextubation 106
Postischemic dysfunction 126
Preoxygenation 106
Pressure 18
   control system 24f
   gauge 26f
   injuries 79
   swing adsorption 6, 12, 32, 43
   plant 3, 4
Pressurized oxygen cylinder 29, 30
Progesterone 84
Pro-inflammatory cytokines 116
Protein-gas binding rate 70
Pseudomonas aeruginosa 101
Pulmonary blood flow 69
Pulmonary capillaries 69
Pulmonary edema 28, 84
Pulmonary embolism 28, 84
Pulmonary function test 116
Pulmonary hypertension 128
Pulmonary shunt 130
Pulmonary toxicity 133
Pulse oximeter
   components of 75
   principle of 75f
   signals 78b
Pulse oximetry 73, 76
   advantages of 76b
   applications of 76

R

Radiation injury, chronic 111
Radio frequency identification 43
Red blood cell 85
Reflectance oximetry 75
Refractory osteomyelitis 111
Renal tubular acidosis 86
Reperfusion injury 126
Reservoir systems 131
Respiratory alkalosis, causes of 84b
Respiratory centre 55
Respiratory drive 57
Respiratory failure 81, 92
Respiratory rate 105

S

Safety regulations 110
Safety system 10, 11
Salicylates 84
Sepsis 78, 136
Shock
   electric 79
   septic 78
Shunt, left-to-right 71
Sickness impact profile score 31
Sinuses 113
Skin
   grafts and flaps 111
   irritation 79
   pigmentation 78
Sleep apnea 106
Stagnant anoxia 61
Stagnant hypoxia 51, 123, 131
Staphylococcus aureus 101
Stationary oxygen concentrator 33f
Stationary unit 25, 26f
   components of 26f
ST-elevation myocardial infarction 134
Stroke 119, 134, 135
Sulfhemoglobin 73
Supplemental oxygen 135
   gradient, effect of 49

T

Thermal injury, acute 112

Tissue oxygenation, measures of 51
Toxic effects 115
Toxins 84
Tracheostomy 99
Transmission oximetry 75
Transtracheal oxygen catheter 94, 95f
Tumor angiogenesis 126
Tyrosine hydroxylase 125

U

Uremia 84
Urinary chloride 85

V

Vacuum 10
   insulated evaporator 24
   pressure swing adsorption plant 3, 4
   system 13
Vacuum-insulated evaporator 24f
Valve service units 8, 9f, 10, 11f
Venous blood gas 80t
Vent valve 26f
Ventilation 58
Venturi devices,
   color-coded 96f
Venturi mask 95, 95f, 96
   functionality 95f
Venturi principle 95f
Volatile acids 82
Vomiting 81

W

Ward vacuum unit 14f
Wound healing 111

Z

Zone valves 10

EU GSPR Authorised Reprsentative
Logos Europe, 9 rue Nicolas Poussin
1700, La Rochelle, France
Phone: +33 (0) 6 67 93 73 78
E-mail: contact@logoseurope.eu

www.ingramcontent.com/pod-product-compliance
Ingram Content Group UK Ltd.
Pitfield, Milton Keynes, MK11 3LW, UK
UKHW050457150426
5217IPUK00025B/1721